Endor

Dream

"David said, 'I will bless ___ ___ counsel; My heart also instructs me in the night seasons'" (Psalm 16:7 NKJV). Although God is faithful to instruct His children, yet far too many fail to understand His instructions because they are usually sealed messages contained in dreams, which must be interpreted. Terri Meredith's *Dreams Revealed* is a balanced, scripturally based book that will help people who long to understand what God is showing them through their dreams. Using both personal examples of her own, as well as biblical dreams, she walks her readers step by step through the interpretation process. Whether one is a just beginning or well experienced in dream interpretation, he or she will find *Dreams Revealed* a helpful resource."
Ira Milligan, President of Servant Ministries, Inc., author of *Understanding the Dreams You Dream, Biblical Keys for Hearing God's Voice in the Night*

"*Dreams Revealed* is an easy-to-read, practical guide to understand how God speaks in dreams. Terri Meredith provides clear and concise wisdom to assist in dream interpretation, which allows the Holy Spirit to amplify His message to the believer. Anyone seeking to hear the voice of the Lord in their dreams would be greatly benefited by reading this book."
Apostle Jane Hamon, senior co-pastor of Vision Church at Christian International and author of *Dreams and Visions: Understanding Your Dreams and How God Can Use Them To Speak To You Today*

"*Dreams Revealed* is a powerful tool to help the dreamer understand how to interpret dreams and visions."
Debora Reeves MSW, LCSW, CADC, author of *Dreams and Visions* and co-owner and therapist at Lighthouse Professional Counseling Services

"God is speaking to you in your dreams. Learn how to understand the messages with *Dreams Revealed*."
Beth Stewart, founder of *Triumphant Living* radio ministry and CEO of Beth Stewart Ministries

"Terri Meredith simplifies the process of decoding the meaning of dreams in this important resource. *Dreams Revealed* is a rock-solid dream interpretation manual."
Sheila Salisbury-Sizemore, instructor, Christian Healing Certification Program, Global Awakening

"This amazing book will help you understand the strange symbolism of the dream world. I am so excited about *Dreams Revealed* and highly recommend it."
Linda Harlow, founder of Kingdom Eagles Ministry, leader of a local dream interpretation ministry, and former owner of a Christian bookstore

"I believe *Dreams Revealed* will bless, encourage, and enlighten many people."
Chuck Lawrence, senior pastor of Christ Temple Church

"I have known Terri over a decade, and I highly recommend *Dreams Revealed* as an excellent resource."
Helen Wolfe, senior pastor of New Day Ministries Church

About the *Dreams Revealed* Series

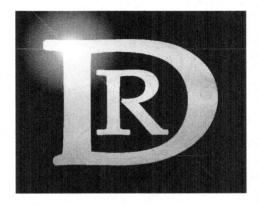

This series comprises tools for learning and growing in dream interpretation.

The Handbook for Biblical Dream Interpretation provides the scientific and spiritual basics of dreaming, explains what to do with dreams when you have them, describes how to interpret dreams, and includes a dream symbol dictionary to help you understand the spiritual meanings behind words.
Hardcover ISBN: 978-1-937331-76-4. Paperback ISBN: 978-1-937331-74-0. e-Book ISBN: 978-1-937331-75-7.

The Expanded Dictionary of Dream Symbols is a comprehensive dream symbol dictionary that contains some of the harder-to-find symbols with their meanings.
Paperback ISBN: 978-1-937331-77-1. e-Book ISBN: 978-1-937331-78-8.

The Personal Dream Journal is a beautiful journal that can be used for capturing dreams and corresponding interpretations.
Paperback ISBN: 978-1-937331-79-5.

DREAMS REVEALED
Handbook for Biblical Dream Interpretation

Terri Meredith

Copyright @ 2014 ShadeTree Publishing, LLC

Dreams Revealed Series ISBN: 978-1-937331-80-1
Hardcover ISBN: 978-1-937331-76-4
Paperback ISBN: 978-1-937331-74-0
e-Book ISBN: 978-1-937331-75-7

Scripture quotations marked NIV are taken from the HOLY BIBLE, NEW INTERNATIONAL VERSION®. Copyright © 1973, 1978, 1984 International Bible Society. Used by permission of Zondervan. All rights reserved.

Scripture quotations marked KJV are taken from the King James Version. The KJV is public domain in the United States.

Scripture quotations marked NKJV are taken from the New King James Version®. Copyright © 1982 by Thomas Nelson, Inc. All rights reserved.

Cover Art by Heather May Photography.

All rights reserved. This book is protected by copyright. No part of this book may be reproduced or transmitted in any form or by any means, electronic or mechanical, including photocopying, recording, or by any information storage and retrieval system, without permission in writing from the publisher.

The purpose of this book is to educate and enlighten. This book is sold with the understanding that the author and publisher are not engaged in rendering counseling, albeit it professional or lay, to the reader or anyone else. The author and publisher shall have neither liability nor responsibility to any person or entity with respect to any loss or damage caused, or alleged to have been caused, directly or indirectly, by the information contained in this book.

Names and details of dreams may have been changed to protect the identity of the dreamer.

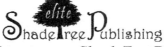

ShadeTree Publishing

Visit our website at www.ShadeTreePublishing.com.

I dedicate this book

To my mother in Heaven, who listened with interest to my dreams and shared in the fascination of watching them come to pass over the years, without once questioning my sanity.

To my Teacher, the Holy Spirit.

To dreamers, that the secret messages in dreams be revealed to you. God bless your journey.

"I, the LORD, reveal myself to them in visions,
I speak to them in dreams" (Numbers 12:6 NIV)

God speaks to us through dreams, but what is He saying?

CONTENTS

List of Tables

List of Figures

PREFACE

On my journey to Jesus some forty years ago, I had a dream that awakened me to my spiritual condition and shook my whole world.

Standing on a sidewalk in my hometown, I could see a white-robed man in the distance and recognized Him as Jesus. I began a brisk walk down the sidewalk toward Him and the group of people around Him. When I finally reached Him, I nearly touched the back of His robe when suddenly He was gone. I asked the group where Jesus went, but they were just as surprised as I was at His disappearance. A couple of the men told me that I was so close, and that I just missed Him. Someone in the group told me that He may have gone to the opposite street corner to speak to another group.

I dashed off in the indicated direction, all the while wondering how I missed Jesus. After a trek that seemed twice as long as the previous one, I finally arrived where He was, only to have Him disappear the moment I arrived. Confused and speechless for a moment, I stood with a group similar to the first. Someone told me I had missed Jesus by only an inch and the group agreed. Running on a now monotonous trek to the opposite corner where Jesus stood,

I was halted by a tremor. I slowed my walking in an attempt to discern the earth's movement while questioning how an earthquake could be happening in this region. I was not prepared for what happened next.

The street began to vibrate, and the vibrations were followed by a violent shaking. I watched helplessly as cars lost control, running into hydrants and buildings. Telephone poles were falling like matchsticks, electric wires dangled, and people were hit by flying debris. Screams filled the air. People were running aimlessly with nowhere to go. The once-quiet city was now in pandemonium. The earth in front of me formed a long jagged seam, which ripped wide open. I watched in horror as those standing near fell into the deep and ever-widening chasm. The earth swallowed people as an open grave. The echoing screams were chilling and horrifying. My next thought was much scarier than the destruction going on around me. *Oh no, it's over... I didn't make it. My time ran out.* It was the most hopeless feeling that I have ever experienced. There were no more chances to reach Jesus. But I was so close...

The sinking feeling I experienced when I awoke (and let me say, I was never so glad to be awake) left me with one fearful question, "Where am I missing Jesus?" The scary fact is, I thought I was fine (sort of).

I became acutely aware that if the Lord would have come that day, I would not have made it into Heaven. Even though preachers were declaring the gospel message all around me, I didn't listen because I thought I was alright and it didn't apply to me. I was the lukewarm Christian scripture talks about, neither hot nor cold. Although I had always gone to church and did the things I knew to do (take communion, attend church events, and even get baptized), I always knew something was missing. Even in my prayer times, God seemed far away. The dream was a warning that I was not ready for the coming of the Lord.

The Lord knew exactly how to reach me, and when I reached back for Him in great desperation, He filled me with His Holy Spirit. Everything changed for me at that moment. (Just as an aside: If you need salvation or to be filled with the Holy Spirit, please spend the next few minutes calling out to Him, repenting of your sins, and praising Him for His goodness and mercy. He longs for you to seek Him.)

With the help of the Holy Spirit, the door to spiritual dreams opened up to me in a greater way. Dreams are now a major part of my life.

I pray this book incites you to take your dreams more seriously, teaches you basic interpretation techniques, and most importantly, impresses upon you that God has more for you and wants to do something amazing in your life. Tonight in your dreams, perhaps He will be telling you about these great plans. Will you be listening?

INTRODUCTION

Dreams are scriptural. God has always spoken through dreams and visions, from Genesis to Revelation and even today. Everyone dreams, and a good portion of our lives is spent dreaming. According to John Paul Jackson, "One-third of the Bible is devoted to dreams, visions, and prophecy, and you will spend one-third of your life asleep. By the time you are sixty years old you will have slept twenty years!"[1] That's a lot of time for the Lord to speak to you.

Often our busy lives keep us so distracted that the best way for us to hear is while sleeping. Dreaming is a time when God has our undivided attention, and He can speak to us, without us talking back or busying ourselves with something else that drowns out His voice. He uses dreams to tell us things about our purpose, prayers, character, and even hidden sin. Many people report receiving creative ideas and inventions in dreams: for example, the invention of the sewing machine by Elias Howell, the song, "Yesterday" written by Paul McCartney, and the song "I Am" written by Eddie James. Solomon received an impartation of the gift of wisdom in a dream.

I realized the importance of dreams in my own life when I started having lots of them. Even though initially I did not have a lot of understanding of dream symbols and language, the dreams just kept coming. In those days, there was not much information on deciphering the meaning of dreams, so I spent many years digging for Christian resources and seeking the Holy Spirit for the ability to understand what my dreams were saying. As I began to understand my dreams, I was then able to start helping others understand their own. Eventually, word of my ability to interpret dreams spread, and I found myself operating in what seemed like a fulltime dream interpretation ministry. When I cried out to the Lord for help, He responded with, "Teach them how to interpret." From that moment on, instead of interpreting dreams for everyone, I began to teach them what I had learned. It seemed like in no time at all, they were understanding their dreams. I wrote this book to share my knowledge and experience of biblical dream interpretation with those who wake up thinking (like I used to), *What on earth was that about?*

This book contains the basic tools and information to get you started understanding your own dreams. Unit 1 contains the scientific and spiritual basics of dreaming. Unit 2 explains what to do with dreams when you have them. Unit 3 describes how to interpret dreams and clearly lays out the steps. Unit 4 is a comprehensive dream symbol dictionary to help you understand the spiritual meanings behind words.

Remember that an incredible amount of information is available to you in dreams if you will tap in to them and get understanding. I believe this book will help you accelerate the learning process of dream interpretation. What took me years of pacing the floors praying, searching the Bible, and examining my dreams, you will now have at your fingertips.

Terri Meredith

This is the book I wish I had thirty years ago. There is an old saying: "Give a man a fish and you have fed him for today. Teach a man to fish and you have fed him for a lifetime." This saying is true with dreamers, and I pray this book feeds your spirit.

UNIT 1:
THE BASICS OF DREAMING

This unit describes the basics of dreaming from both a scientific and a biblical point of reference.

THE SCIENCE OF SLEEP

Knowing the science behind sleep helps us to understand how sleep and dreams are physically important and how we can use the knowledge to get the best sleep possible, thereby increasing our ability to dream.

Much of what we know about sleep is via polysomnography, which are studies that record brain waves, the oxygen level in the blood, heart rate, and breathing, as well as eye and leg movements during sleep. Using these types of studies, scientists have determined that we sleep in five distinct stages and that dreaming occurs predominately in one of them. In addition, the scientists were able to derive recommendations for the appropriate amount of sleep people should get each night.

Five Stages of Sleep

The first four stages of sleep are classified as NREM (Non-Rapid Eye Movement) and the last stage is known as REM (Rapid Eye Movement). Each stage of sleep serves a distinct purpose. You may cycle through the five stages of sleep four to six times per night, not necessarily in the same order once you go through the initial stages. It is common to begin again in Stage 2 (because your body is already rested) and then progress from there.

The latter half of sleep is more dominated by REM sleep while the first half of the night is dominated by slow-wave sleep. Adults spend about 50 percent of their sleep in Stage 2, 20 percent in REM, and the other 30 percent moving between the remaining three stages. Older adults often spend less time in REM sleep while younger children spend about half of their sleep in REM. Lack of REM sleep can impair the ability to learn complex tasks.[2]

Stage One

In this stage, the dreamer is dozing off or "half asleep". Because the muscles are still active while the sleeper is drifting, the sleeper may twitch and is easily awakened. The eyes roll slowly and may open and close at times. The brain waves in this stage are classified as theta waves (see Figure 1). There may be a few minutes of dreaming; however, subjects who wake in this stage generally describe their dream more as random thoughts rather than a dream. The duration of Stage 1 lasts only five to ten minutes while the body relaxes.

Stage Two

In this stage of sleep, it becomes gradually harder to wake, and the eyes stop moving. Body temperature drops, making a cooler environment more pleasurable for sleep. The theta waves continue and are interrupted by abrupt brain activity called sleep spindles and K complexes (see Figure 1).

Stages Three and Four

In these stages, the sleeper is less responsive to environmental noises and movement, and breathing slows. Sleepwalking and talking predominately occur during this time. In terms of brain waves, these stages are referred to as slow-wave sleep, wherein the brain waves decrease in frequency and become delta waves (see Figure 1). There is no real division between Stages 3 and 4 except that in Stage 3, delta waves are typically less than half of the amount of brain waves, whereas in Stage 4, delta waves are more than half.

REM Sleep

In this stage of sleep, the eyes begin to move rapidly, hence the name of the stage. The brain releases chemicals signaling the paralysis of limb muscles to prevent voluntary muscle movement and lessen the chance of the dreamer hurting him or herself while dreaming.

This stage of sleep is also referred to as paradoxical sleep. The paradox is that, while brain waves are similar to waking sleep during this stage (see Figure 1), the sleeper is harder to arouse than in any other sleep stage. Brain waves are similar to those in the awake state and show that the brain is more active than when awake.

REM sleep occurs about ninety minutes into sleep and is when most dreams occur (as a result of heightened brain activity). The first period of REM usually lasts around ten minutes, with each recurring REM stage lengthening; the final one may last up to sixty minutes.[3] With a full night's sleep, a person could go through three to five intervals of REM.

Figure 1. Examples of Brain Wave Activity During Wake and Sleep

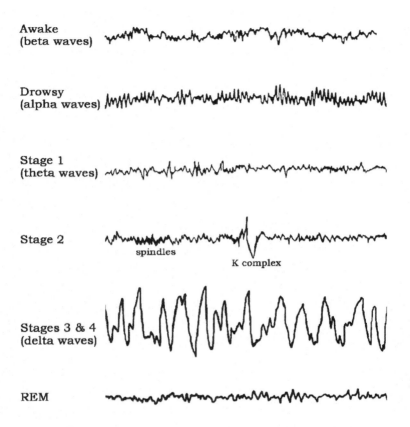

The Science of Dreams

Our Creator made us to sleep and to dream. Even though some people claim they do not dream, science indicates that we all dream approximately three to five dreams per night, up to seven in some cases, with a full night's sleep.[4]

Sleep cycles play a role in our dreams. Some theories call the early stages of sleep a dreamless sleep; others say it is a light sleep with a few minutes of dreaming. Dreams are not usually memorable or vivid until you get into this stage. The longer you sleep, the more time you have in REM sleep because the length of time spent dreaming in REM increases gradually throughout the night, with the longest REM sleep occurring just before you wake up.

In an early sleep study by the University of Chicago's Sleep Research Laboratory, when subjects were awakened during REM sleep, twenty of twenty-seven people (74 percent) recalled vivid dreams. When awakened in NREM sleep, only four of twenty-three people (17 percent) recalled having a dream.[5]

If you wake up while in REM, you can jot down the main points of your dream and go right back into REM sleep. Some people set an alarm every 90 to 120 minutes to capture their dreams while in REM sleep. (Personally, I value my sleep too much to purposefully interrupt it.)

If you sleep all the way through the night, you may only remember your last dream. However, I know people who recall multiple dreams each night. For myself, I may recall two or three dreams per night. So how do I do this? When I exit REM and return back to the beginning stages of sleep, I am able to regain consciousness long enough to recall the dream before slipping into deeper sleep.

Your best dreaming time is right before you awaken in the morning, because the last stage of REM sleep may last up to sixty minutes and provide long periods of uninterrupted dreaming.[6] This may help us to understand why some dreamers have long, epic dreams, and sometimes feel like they dreamed a particular dream all night. The important thing to remember is that nothing God gives is wasted. A dream lasting only a minute could give you the answer you have been praying for.

Anyone who has ever been able to recall a dream knows how illogical they can be. The frontal cortex of the brain is where logic and reasoning are processed. During sleep, there is decreased brain activity in this region, causing the possible and impossible to fuse in dreams. When our dreams are illogical or we are performing impossible acts (i.e., flying or breathing underwater), this physiological phenomenon allows the dreamer to continue without waking up to question the logic.[7]

A special kind of dreaming, called lucid dreaming, occurs in a small number of people. During lucid dreaming, you become aware that you are dreaming without waking from the dream. You may (but not always) consciously interact with the dream or have some control over your actions in it. In one of my lucid dreams, I was watching my dream take place while standing to the side interpreting it as it was happening. When I realized that I needed to stop and let the dream finish, I could no longer see myself.

Lucid dreaming is a hybrid-like state of sleep with features of both REM sleep (delta and theta brain waves) and waking (gamma brain waves). In order to move from non-lucid REM sleep dreaming to lucid REM sleep dreaming, the brain activity shifts toward waking.[8] As a result, the frontal regions of the brain become more active and thus promote lucid insight into the dream state and control of your actions.

One of the benefits of lucid dreaming is that dreamers can overcome fears in their dreams. Rather than allowing an attack, they are able to stand up to it and overcome it while in the dream state.

Sleep Recommendations

According to the National Sleep Foundation, our sleep needs depend on age, lifestyle, and health. In 2015, the foundation provided new guidelines on the amount of sleep needed per age group. They recommend, in general, seven to nine hours of sleep for healthy adults (ages 18 to 64 years). Younger children require more sleep, while older adults (65+ years) require slightly less.[9]

Shaving even a little time off sleep can have a negative short-term and long-term effect on health. In a National Sleep Foundation survey of Americans, forty-five percent of responders reported that poor or insufficient sleep had affected their daily activities at least once in the past seven days.[10]

Lack of sleep can cause a breakdown in cognitive functions, decreased performance, and daytime sleepiness. A common reaction following many sleepless nights is crying because there is a decreased ability to handle stress. Staying up late into the early morning hours has been associated with obesity, high blood pressure, and a host of other illnesses.

Too little (and too much) sleep has been associated with a higher death rate. The American Cancer Society conducted a survey in 1.1 million men and women from 30 to 102 years of age.[11] Participants who reported sleeping six or less hours (and eight or more hours) had a higher death rate.

Statistics show that 62 percent of American adults experience problems sleeping a few nights per week, and forty million Americans have sleep disorders.[12] The growing industry of clinics, sleep aids, pills, medical services, devices, and other related sleep services was expected to surpass thirty-two billion dollars.[13]

The best way to improve sleep is to follow the sleep recommendations as often as possible. However, this in itself may not be enough. Despite sleeping within the recommended number of hours a night, 35 percent of Americans reported their sleep quality as "poor" or "only fair," and 20 percent reported that they did not wake up feeling refreshed in the previous seven days.[14] In general, this sleep quality was highly associated with the participants' overall health, as 67 percent of those with less than good sleep quality also reported "poor" or "only fair" health. In addition, low life satisfaction and high stress were also related to poor sleep quality.

Other than decreasing stress and improving health, there are additional measures someone can take to improve sleep. According to Dr. Oz, the best time to go to sleep is before 11 p.m. and the best time to wake is 6:30 a.m. or sunrise;[15] so, if you are used to being a night owl, you may consider retraining your internal clock. Furthermore, it is best to sleep in a cool, very dark room. Before bedtime, avoid lighted screens (e.g., TV, computer, and cell phones), large meals, alcohol, caffeine, and other stimulants (e.g., nicotine).

One reason people are not dreaming well is that they are not sleeping well. Following the recommended guidelines for better sleep will do wonders for your overall health as well as your dream life.

THE SOURCE OF YOUR DREAMS

The source of our dreams forms the predominant line existing between psychological-based versus Bible-based interpretation of dreams. One contends that dreams only arise from internal mechanisms in the individual, while the other asserts that dreams also come from external sources like God.

The psychological view of dreams tends to look at the source of dreams coming from within the subconscious mind, dealing with inner conflicts and imbalances. Some psychological models tend to focus on unresolved childhood issues and the inner-self as our god.

Sigmund Freud (1856–1939) talked heavily on the subject of sexual impulses from childhood that are dealt with later as an adult because the young mind could not process or understand them at the time. The Freudian view is based on fulfilling desires that are related to childhood memories and experiences. In particular, dreams are thought to reveal issues stemming from the dreamer's childhood relationship with his or her mother.

Carl Jung (1875–1960), the founder of analytical psychology and a key figure in the development of the New Age movement, alleged that dreams were manifestations of unresolved emotional conflicts and imbalances in our male/female nature. Jung eventually split from Freud, rejecting the idea that dreams are related to sexual impulses. In *A Psychological Approach to the Doctrine of the Trinity*,[16] Jung perverts the concept of the Trinity by claiming that 1) God the Father is the self and the source of energy within the psyche, 2) the Son is a consciousness that replaces the ego, and 3) the Holy Spirit is a mediator between the ego and the self. Jung wrote a number of books and articles about Eastern religions, including commentaries on the *Tibetan Book of the Dead*, yoga, and Eastern meditation. He also contributed forewords to books including *Introduction to Zen Buddhism, Holy Men of India*, and the *I Ching*.[17]

Most secular teachings solely focus on the subconscious mind, inner emotions, and feelings when it comes to dreams. While these types of dreams (often referred to as "soul dreams" in biblical dream interpretation) certainly exist, there are other sources of dreams outside of ourselves. Basically, our dreams can come from our soul (i.e., mind, will, emotions, and flesh), the enemy, or God.

When considering dream interpretation models, it is important to remember the story of how King Saul became so desperate for answers that he sought them through witchcraft instead of godly methods (see 1 Samuel 28:6). Not only was he later rebuked, but he received a promise of death. This story tells us that we need to be very careful about dream interpretation models that exclude God. And if that is not enough, consider the Lord's warning to not listen to diviners who are not from Him.[18]

Dreams from the Soul

Because soul dreams come from our mind, will, emotions, and/or flesh, and lack the spiritual connection you have with God, they do not come bearing heavenly messages for interpretation. However, these dreams are not completely useless to us because they can reveal the status of our heart and intentions, and reveal sin in our lives. Do not be too hasty discarding them until you mine them for possible gold.

When something is on our mind or is repetitive in our life, it can show up in dreams. In today's society, busyness and preoccupation run rampant through the lives of many people. The things that consume us during the day, including the things we set forth with our own words, can haunt us in the night. The Bible says that "a dream cometh through the multitude of business; and a fool's voice is known by multitude of words."[19] When we have these sorts of mind-driven dreams, we need to ask ourselves what is occupying our mind, especially in the places that should be filled with thoughts toward God.

Sometimes our will for something can be so strong, and almost obsessive, that it can affect our dreams. Probably the most common dreams that are brought on by our desires are sexual ones. While some sexual dreams are healthy and not sinful (for example, dreaming of relations with a spouse), most sexual dreams reveal unresolved and lingering sin in our lives. Regardless of the nature of the will-driven dream, it can provide information as to what our hearts are set upon. After all, where your treasure is, there your heart will be also.[20]

Emotions are a very powerful force for causing dreams. For example, when my sister passed away at an early age, I was filled with extreme sorrow over her untimely death. For weeks, I dreamed nearly every night about her. The dreams were strange; they did not flow from scene to scene, but instead, were fragmented, like a puzzle with pieces missing. She was often in her casket or lying in a bed sleeping. As time went by, the dreams eased up and eventually stopped. I understood throughout the entire process that I was working through a deep grief. Although emotion-driven dreams can be overwhelming, they can reveal feelings that the dreamer needs to deal with.

Dreams caused by our flesh are brought on by things such as hunger, drugs, or pregnancy. Once while I was fasting and praying, I dreamed I was eating fresh, hot, delicious pizza. This was a dream straight from my hungry soul. Drugs and alcohol have multiple pathways for influencing our dreams. They can directly affect our brain or interfere with our sleep cycles (especially REM). Many medications, especially anesthesia, can induce crazy dreams. Have you ever heard of someone coming out of anesthesia picking at imaginary bugs or something equally bizarre? Pregnancy is interesting because not only do the mother's hormones affect her dreams, but also, the baby itself does. After about seven months into development, the baby starts to dream, and many women report a change in their own dreams as a result.

Dreams from the Enemy

Make no mistake about it—your enemy, the devil, is prowling around like a roaring lion looking to devour you.[21]

It does not matter whether we are awake or asleep, his quest is relentless.

Dreams from the enemy have telltale signs. Oftentimes, they are dark, without color or light, and drenched with fear-evoking images and experiences. Many times after these sorts of dreams, the dreamer is left feeling intense negative emotions and/or like he has been "slimed". The aftereffects of the dream are directly associated with the initial purpose of it.

You have a destiny and a God-given purpose on the earth, and the enemy will do everything possible to make you to believe otherwise. He can't stop you, but he will speak lies to keep you from believing the truth of what God says about you. The Bible says that while everyone was sleeping, his enemy came and sowed weeds among the wheat.[22] He sows lies among the truth to scare you, get you off your path, separate you from God, and get you into bondage.

Scripture says to draw near to God, and He will draw near to you.[23] But did you know this can work with the enemy, too? If we draw near to the enemy, he will drawer near to us.

Before evil can enter our life, it must first have a door. When you watch, read, or listen to dark material, you open doors to allow evil influences into your life. Not long after "vampire romance" books and movies debuted, young girls came to me with dreams about vampires chasing them, trying to bite them, or turning their friends into other vampires. Before commenting on their dream, I first asked whether they were watching vampire movies or reading the books. (The answer was nearly always yes.) I explained the dream to them and cautioned them about continuing to entertain themselves with the blood lore. I explained that vampires crave blood, and how opening the door to this bloodlust can later manifest in cutting, harming oneself, or romanticizing death.

Some people deliberately open themselves up for dark dreams and welcome them. Stephen King (horror novelist) finds inspiration for his novels in dreams. In an interview with Stan Nicholls, King discussed his inspiration for *Misery* that came through a dream.[24]

The enemy can influence your dreams, especially if you are involved in willful, open sin of any kind. For instance, when a dreamer is involved in the occult, the enemy has open access to his or her life. Other examples are lust of the flesh, which can cause X-rated dreams, and bitterness, which can cause dreams about hurting people.

More than likely, after having an enemy dream, you will spend a lot of effort trying to get it out of your mind. However, do not discard them too hastily because they can reveal the enemy's perception of your weaknesses and his plans of attack on your life. Pray that the Holy Spirit will help you close and lock any open doors in your life.

Dreams from God

When God created man, He created within him the ability to dream. While our prayer life is the time we spend speaking to the Father, our dream life is a time when He speaks to us. It is God the Father, through His Holy Spirit, who is the Giver and the Interpreter of God-inspired dreams.

Dreams are like fresh manna of revelation, so to speak, that is new every morning. Just like the reaction of the

Israelites to the manna, our reaction to our dreams may be, "What is it?" Because alone in our own knowledge and wisdom, we cannot understand the mind of God, we need the help of the Holy Spirit to discern the meaning of our dreams. The Bible says that a "person without the Spirit does not accept the things that come from the Spirit of God but considers them foolishness, and cannot understand them because they are discerned only through the Spirit."[25] Dreams are just one more way God causes us to seek Him.

God has many practical reasons for speaking to us in dreams. It is a time when we must listen and cannot talk back or rebut. Because the enemy is not omnipotent like God, he cannot read our thoughts, and therefore, he does not have ears or eyes on the "conversation." With the quickly approaching end of days, it is even more imperative that people can glean instructions from the Lord, and is probably why the Bible says that dreams will increase in the last days.[26]

In general, dreams from God are rich with color, full of symbolism, and congruent with His character and Word. It is important to understand, though, that God is not limited to these dream attributes. It may be tempting to think a black-and-white dream is from the enemy, when in reality, God is speaking to you about discernment in an issue with no room for gray areas. God-given dreams may include situations that are familiar to you, and yet will cause you to seek deeper understanding. They necessitate revelation and interpretation from a heavenly perspective.

The Lord's desire is for us to learn what He is saying. Through dreams, He prepares us mentally and emotionally for many situations that will arise. He calls us into intercession and prayer for others and ourselves, and warns us of impending danger or evil. God uses dreams as lessons and revelation that will stretch our thinking in new ways. He can even heal us of physical, emotional, or psychological trauma while in a dream. Not all dreams from God are positive, and not all negative dreams are from the enemy. Sometimes God may rebuke us for unresolved sin in our lives. Even when dreams seem negative, they can still bring hope and strategy to a potentially bad situation.

Many dreams have more meaning to them than we think. As you train your spiritual senses to recognize a dream from the Lord, it is the most wonderful experience to get revelation in this way. Over the years, I have learned to recognize dreams from God and trust the revelation they imparted. I pray that over time you will see dreams unfold in your life, too.

COMMON TYPES OF DREAMS

Dreams can be supernatural (above the natural intellect) and prophetic (revelation from God). They come in two varieties, literal or symbolic, and can even be a mix of both. When the Lord has an urgent message with little tolerance for error in understanding (like life-or-death situations), He tends to give very literal dreams. However, for most circumstances, He uses symbolic dreams. While you may be praying for literal or simpler dreams instead of symbolic ones that take more work to understand, you need to know that when much is given, much is required.[27] Your accountability for understanding and correctly reacting to the dream skyrockets with literal dreams.

The five most common types of dreams are
1) Literal
2) Prophetic
3) Direction/Calling
4) Warning
5) Dark

Other types exist including dreams of confirmation, rebuke, and spiritual cleansing. In general, though, all dreams have a component of intercession, and should always incite prayer.

Literal Dreams

On first consideration, many dreamers believe their dreams are literal because they fail to understand how God uses symbolism to speak to us, and literal dreams require little or no interpretation. In general, if everything in the dream appears as it does in real life, then it usually can be taken literally; however, if even one thing seems unrealistic, then the possibility that the entire dream is symbolic must be considered.

Literal dreams can have a prophetic aspect for future events and thus be a very serious call to intercession. Several times, I have dreamed of a literal catastrophic or world event that later appeared in the news. For example, in 2004, I dreamed of the tsunami that occurred in Indonesia. In the dream I was walking around a beach area observing the people. I strode around a corner passing a white billboard before heading to a nearby building in a town running parallel to the beach. As I made my way to the third floor overlooking the ocean, I could see through every window. When I looked out over the Indian Ocean, I saw a huge watery eruption rising and coming toward the shore. Running to the ground toward the beach, I tried to warn the people, but I only made it to the billboard at the entrance of the beach. The huge wave washed over the billboard and building, and was ready to wash over where I was standing when I awoke. In real life, when I saw the story on the news, the white billboard, hotel, and town were all exactly how I saw it in the dream. The newscaster stood in front of the sign reporting the disaster and the estimated 230,000 deaths.

Ten days prior to his assassination, Abraham Lincoln dreamed of a death. In the dream he heard sobs and mourning. He saw a corpse wrapped up and being guarded in the east wing of the White House, and when he asked who it was, the reply was "the president." Lincoln's dream was not symbolic, and everything about it appeared literal. The only unknown was the timing of the future event. I wonder, if he had understood the importance of this dream, could he have changed his plans and avoided his assassination. This is a great illustration of the greater accountability and urgency associated with literal dreams.

You may not know whether your dream is literal or symbolic until it occurs, but I realized the day I saw the tsunami newscast that I did not pray hard or long enough. You may wonder what the point of prayer is when a tragedy happens anyway. I believe that it is still important to pray, and I oftentimes focus prayers for people to make decisions, to leave the region, to find a protected place, or most importantly, to receive the gospel message.

Prophetic Dreams

Prophetic dreams always reveal an aspect of a future event or outcome. These types of dreams occur on occasion in the average dreamers to forewarn them of an upcoming event in their life. Because these dreams occur infrequently, they can prove to be difficult for the dreamer to interpret.

A handful of Christians have been appointed by God as official prophetic dreamers. These dreamers are designated watchmen for the Kingdom. They may serve at an international, national, or local level. Because they are appointed by God, He makes sure they have the ear of kings, presidents, or pastors. Many of these watchmen work under the radar and without public affirmation and acknowledgment.

Direction/Calling Dreams

Direction dreams give insight on how to approach or handle a situation. God uses this type of dream to prune us and guide us into the near future. In addition, He may use a direction dream to rebuke us for our previous bad actions and instruct us on how to make amends.

Calling dreams point us to the path of our vocation or calling in life. In these dreams, we may see ourselves doing certain things or performing tasks that we are not necessarily doing at the time. Generally, the action is associated with gifts, talents, and passions that we possess. Although direction and calling dreams sound very similar, the main difference is that direction dreams tend to deal with our next step, while calling dreams address our entire path ahead.

Warning Dreams

Warning dreams prepare us for something that can possibly be avoided. We always hope to derive a positive meaning from our dreams, but when a warning is issued, it is important to pay special attention. These dreams alert us to potential danger or harm; they should not make us fearful, but instead, ready to put on the armor of God and fight.

Probably the hardest warning dreams to swallow are the ones warning us to straighten up and change our ways. The dream may come with harsh prophetic consequences to get our attention. In addition, if we do not heed the warning the first time, God will continue to bombard us with more dreams that may seem different, but carry the same message.

Dark Dreams

Dark dreams are nearly always described as nightmares and involve a great deal of fear. They can entail death of a loved one, phobias, being chased, or other fear-based themes. For example, a man who had a fear of public speaking in real life kept having dreams that he could not speak or scream.

The enemy thrives on fear as a tool to hold us back. Although dark dreams are very undesirable, they can shed light on fears that we need to face in real life. For example, a monster chasing us could mean we are afraid of something catching up to us. Falling off a cliff and not being able to scream could mean we feel like we have no control and no voice over our circumstances.

Children often have fear-based dreams. It would be just like the enemy to cause children to fear having dreams when they are young and cut off that form of communication from God for their future. Parents need to understand what is happening in the child's life in order to calm them and teach them how to face their fears.

Trauma can bring on dark dreams, too. For example, some dreamers have drowning dreams, especially when dealing with overwhelming situations.

While most dark dreams are from the enemy or born out of our fears or trauma, sometimes God will allow a dark dream to get His point across after we have habitually ignored His previous warnings or instructions.

DREAMS IN THE BIBLE

Dreams were given to people in the Old and New Testaments, to the righteous and the heathen. Piecing biblical dreams together helps us paint a larger prophetic picture than the dreamers could have possibly imagined at the time.

Dreams were a commonly accepted form of revelation in Bible times. When a dream was shared, no one seemed surprised. Today, we might brush it off as a "pizza" dream or diminish its value saying, "Oh, it was just a dream." In our culture, Christians tend to have mixed feelings about them because the concept of dreams has been tainted quite a bit by false teachings. However, like people from the Bible times, we need to understand the importance of dreams and recognize them as a means for God to speak to us.

Dreamers throughout the Bible wanted to know the meaning of their dreams. They placed a high value on them and followed through when applicable. Because in the Old Testament times, Jesus had not yet come and the Holy Spirit was not yet released after His crucifixion, revelation was precious in those days. Our dreams today often confirm to us what the Holy Spirit has already been showing us or make us aware of something for which we need greater understanding.

From biblical dreams we can learn so much. It is apparent that nothing goes unnoticed by God. He knows the thoughts and intents of every heart. He often spoke into the destiny of a person rather than where they were at a moment in time. For example, Joseph was dreaming he was a ruler when he was seventeen years old, but he didn't rule as prime minister in Egypt until he was thirty. God sees the end from the beginning.

A look at dreams in the Bible provides insight into the profound ways God uses them to set events in place for His people. The dreams listed here are a partial list that excludes trances, visions, and prophetic revelations.

Table 1. A Summary of Biblical Dreams and Their Interpretation

Dream Info	Actual Dream	Interpretation and Significance
Abraham Genesis 15:12–15 Type: prophetic Notes: First recorded dream in the Bible	The Lord told Abraham that his descendants would be a stranger in a land not theirs and that they would be enslaved there for four hundred years. He also said that eventually He would punish the nation enslaving them and Abraham's descendants would come out with great possessions and wealth. He told Abraham that he would die in peace at an old age and the fourth generation of his descendants would come back.	**Interpretation**: This is a prophetic dream of which the interpretation is literal. **Significance**: The events of the dream occurred and were recorded as prophesied.
Abimelech Genesis 20:3–7 Type: warning	God told Abimelech in a dream that he was as good as dead because the woman he took (Abraham's wife) was a married woman. He told Abimelech to return the woman and have Abraham pray for him so that he might live.	**Interpretation**: The dream was a literal warning from God. **Significance**: Because of the dream, Sarah was safeguarded, for she was to be the mother of nations. Also, the dream is proof that God speaks to the unsaved through dreams.

Dreams Revealed:
Handbook for Biblical Dream Interpretation

Dream Info	Actual Dream	Interpretation and Significance
Jacob Genesis 28:11–15 Type: prophetic/calling Notes: Jacob's Ladder	Jacob had a dream he saw a stairway resting on the earth, its top reaching to heaven. Angels of God were ascending and descending on it. Above it stood the Lord, who reaffirmed the Abrahamic covenant with Jacob.	**Interpretation**: This was a literal dream in which the Lord spoke to Jacob and reaffirmed the Abrahamic covenant with him. **Significance**: The dream gave Jacob the encouragement he needed to hold tight the covenant that the Lord made with his father and him.
Jacob Genesis 31:10–13 Type: direction	Jacob had a dream in which the angel of the Lord instructed Jacob how to breed the animals and told him to return to his native land.	**Interpretation**: This dream was literal and showed Jacob how to breed the animals in order to obtain wealth and instructed him to leave Laban and return to his native land. **Significance**: By following the instructions, Jacob became wealthy and was able to leave with a fortune and the finest herds.
Jacob Genesis 46:2–4 Type: direction	God spoke to Jacob in a dream and told him to not fear going to Egypt because He would go with Jacob and make him a great nation there. God also promised to bring him out again.	**Interpretation**: This dream was literal and told Jacob to move to Egypt and live there for a while. **Significance**: Because he heard from God, Jacob packed up his whole family

Dream Info	Actual Dream	Interpretation and Significance
		and moved them to Egypt, thus initiating the fulfillment of the prophecy given to Abraham.
Laban Genesis 31:24 Type: warning	When Laban was pursuing Jacob, God came to Laban in a dream and told him to be careful not to say anything to Jacob, either good or bad.	**Interpretation**: This was a literal dream in which the Lord spoke to Laban. **Significance**: Once Laban caught up with Jacob, the meeting was positive because of the dream. The two men came to an agreement and made a covenant.
Men in Enemy Camp Judges 7:13–15 Type: warning/ prophetic	After sneaking into the enemy's camp, Gideon overheard one of the men telling another about his dream. He saw a round loaf of barley bread tumbling into the Midianite camp and striking the tent with such force that the tent overturned and collapsed.	**Interpretation**: This was a symbolic dream in which the barley bread symbolized Gideon's army, who would overtake the camp. **Significance**: The dream served two purposes: 1) It was a warning to the enemy army that they would fail. 2) It was meant to be overheard by Gideon to increase his faith. When Gideon heard the dream and its interpretation, he led his army to victory.

Dreams Revealed:
Handbook for Biblical Dream Interpretation

Dream Info	Actual Dream	Interpretation and Significance
Joseph Genesis 37:5–6 Type: calling/prophetic	Joseph dreamed that he and his brothers were binding sheaves of grain out in the field when suddenly Joseph's sheaf rose and stood upright, while the brothers' sheaves gathered around his and bowed down to it.	**Interpretation**: This was a symbolic and prophetic dream in which the sheaves of grain represented the brothers bowing down to Joseph. **Significance**: The dream helped to set into motion the events that would lead to its fulfillment. In the end, Jacob's brothers did bow down to him in Egypt.
Joseph Genesis 37:9 Type: calling/prophetic Notes: Confirmed his first dream	Joseph dreamed that the sun and moon and eleven stars were bowing down to him.	**Interpretation**: This was a symbolic and prophetic dream in which the sun and eleven stars represented Joseph's parent(s) and brothers bowing down to him. **Significance**: The dream helped to set into motion the events that would lead to its fulfillment. In the end, Jacob's family did bow down to him in Egypt.
Pharaoh's Cupbearer Genesis 40:9–11 Type: prophetic	In the cupbearer's dream, he saw a vine in front of him. It had three branches, and as soon as it budded, it blossomed, and its clusters ripened into grapes. Then Pharaoh's cup was	**Interpretation**: This was a symbolic and prophetic dream in which the three branches represented three days, after which time the royal cupbearer would be restored to his position.

Dream Info	Actual Dream	Interpretation and Significance
	in the cupbearer's hand, and he took the grapes, squeezed them into the cup, and put the cup in Pharaoh's hand.	**Significance**: The cupbearer was restored in three days as the dream indicated. Also, by Joseph interpreting the dream, it revealed that he was gifted to do so. Years later, the cupbearer remembered Joseph when Pharaoh was in need of a dream interpreter. Not only was Joseph able to help Pharaoh understand his dreams, it was the door of opportunity that allowed Joseph to be elevated in the service of Pharaoh.
Pharaoh's Baker Genesis 40:16–18 Type: prophetic	In the baker's dream, on his head were three baskets of bread. In the top basket were all kinds of baked goods for Pharaoh, but the birds were eating them out of the basket.	**Interpretation**: This was a symbolic and prophetic dream in which the three baskets represented three days, after which time the royal baker would be beheaded. **Significance**: The baker was beheaded in three days as the dream indicated. Also, this served as additional evidence to the royal cupbearer that Joseph was gifted to interpret dreams.

Dream Info	Actual Dream	Interpretation and Significance
Pharaoh Genesis 41:1–4 Type: warning/prophetic Notes: Joseph interpreted Pharaoh's dream	In Pharaoh's dream he was standing on the bank of the Nile, when out of the river came seven fat cows that grazed among the reeds. After them, came seven scrawny cows. The scrawny cows ate the seven fat cows, and afterward, no one could tell that they had done so because they looked just as scrawny as before.	**Interpretation**: This was a symbolic and prophetic dream in which the seven fat cows represented seven years of plenty, while seven scrawny cows represented seven years of famine that would consume the seven years of plenty. **Significance**: Pharaoh received the interpretation and placed Joseph in charge of the land to prepare for the coming famine. The fulfillment of the dream occurred when famine took over the land, and because Joseph was now in a position to help his family, he brought them to Egypt, where they would prosper, yet eventually be enslaved there for four hundred years as indicated in Abraham's prophetic dream.
Pharaoh Genesis 41:5–7; 25–31 Type: confirmation	In Pharaoh's dream he saw seven plump heads of grain growing on a single stalk. After them, seven thin heads of grain sprouted. The thin	**Interpretation**: This was a symbolic and prophetic dream in which the seven plump heads of grain represented seven years of plenty, while seven thin ones

Dream Info	Actual Dream	Interpretation and Significance
Notes: Confirmed his first dream about the cows	heads of grain swallowed up the seven good heads.	represented seven years of famine that would consume the seven years of plenty. **Significance**: This dream directly followed the dream of the fat and scrawny cows. The dream was given to Pharaoh in two forms because the matter had been firmly decided by God, and God would do it soon.
Nebuchadnezzar and Daniel (the same dream given to both) Daniel 2:31–43 Type: prophetic Notes: Daniel received Nebuchadnezzar's dream in a dream and understood the interpretation.	Daniel saw the king's dream of the enormous statue with a head of gold, chest and arms of silver, belly and thighs of bronze, legs of iron, feet of iron/clay. A rock, not cut out by hands, struck the statue and the metals were broken in pieces, the wind swept all of it away, but the rock became a mountain that filled the whole earth	**Interpretation**: This was a symbolic and prophetic dream describing the kingdoms to come after Nebuchadnezzar (the head of gold). The fourth kingdom, as strong as iron, would arise and crush all the others. The following kingdom would be divided, yet have some strength. The final kingdom (God's) would crush all former kingdoms and endure forever. **Significance**: The dream provides a prophecy of the earthly kingdoms that will precede the Kingdom of God. There

Dreams Revealed:
Handbook for Biblical Dream Interpretation

Dream Info	Actual Dream	Interpretation and Significance
		are several eschatological theories on what layers represent which kingdoms.
Nebuchadnezzar Daniel 4:10–17 Type: warning/prophetic	Nebuchadnezzar saw a tree standing before him. The tree was large and strong; its top touched the sky and it was visible to the ends of the earth. It provided food and shelter for the birds and animals. Then he saw coming down from heaven a holy messenger who said to cut down the tree, strip off its leaves, scatter its fruit, and let the stump and its roots, bound with iron and bronze, remain in the ground. The messenger said to let Nebuchadnezzar be drenched with the dew of heaven, let him live with the animals among the plants of the earth, and let him be given the mind of an animal for seven years.	**Interpretation**: This was a symbolic and prophetic dream. The enormous tree represented King Nebuchadnezzar and his power and authority in the earth. The Lord decreed that the king would lose his mind and become as a wild animal until he acknowledged that God is over all the kingdoms of the world and He gives them to whom He wishes. The stump of the tree with its roots symbolized that the kingdom would be later restored. **Significance**: Despite counseling by Daniel, Nebuchadnezzar continued to exalt himself and declare his majesty. However, just as the Lord decreed, a year later, he lost his mind for seven years and literally lived like an animal until he finally acknowledged the Lord. Afterward, his sanity and kingdom were

Dream Info	Actual Dream	Interpretation and Significance
		restored, and Nebuchadnezzar praised and glorified the King of heaven.
Solomon 1 Kings 3:4–15 Type: bestowing of a gift	Following Solomon's sacrifice of a thousand burnt offerings at Gibeon, the Lord appeared to him in dream and instructed him to ask for whatever he desired. Solomon asked for a discerning heart to govern His people and to distinguish between right and wrong.	**Interpretation**: This dream was literal and a visitation from the Lord. **Significance**: Solomon's response pleased the Lord because he did not ask for a long life, wealth, or the death of his enemies; but instead, discernment to administer justice. The Lord gave him a wise and discerning heart. He also gave what he did not ask for, namely wealth and honor, and told him that if he walked in obedience then he would have a long life.
Joseph Matthew 1:20 Type: direction	After Joseph learned about Mary's pregnancy, an angel of the Lord appeared to him in a dream and told him not to be afraid to take her as his wife, because what was conceived in her was from the Holy Spirit. The angel told him that Mary would give birth to a Son, who should be named	**Interpretation**: This dream was literal and a visitation from an angel. **Significance**: Joseph woke up and did as the angel commanded by marrying Mary. Joseph and Mary never consummated their marriage before Jesus' birth; thus, the prophecy was fulfilled about the Savior being born of a

Dream Info	Actual Dream	Interpretation and Significance
	Jesus, and He would save His people from their sins.	virgin. Mary gave birth to Jesus, the Savior of all mankind.
The Magi/Wise Men Matthew 2:12 Type: warning	After presenting their gifts to Jesus, the wise men had a dream in which they were warned not to return to Herod.	**Interpretation**: This dream could have been literal or it could have been symbolic and all that was recorded in the Bible was the interpretation. **Significance**: The wise men did not return the way they came and found their way back to their country by another route.
Joseph Matthew 2:13 Type: warning	After the departure of the wise men, an angel appeared to Joseph in a dream and told him to get up, take the child and his mother and escape to Egypt, and stay there until told otherwise because Herod was going to search for the child to kill him.	**Interpretation**: This dream was literal and a visitation from an angel. **Significance**: Joseph left during the night. In the meantime, Herod was angry with the Magi for not returning to him and ordered all the boys in the area who were two years old and younger to be killed. Because Joseph was obedient, Jesus was not harmed. The family stayed in Egypt until Herod died.

Dream Info	Actual Dream	Interpretation and Significance
Joseph Matthew 2:19–20 Type: direction	After Herod died, an angel appeared to Joseph in a dream and told him to get up and take the child and his mother to the land of Israel, because those who were trying to take the child's life were dead.	**Interpretation**: This dream was literal and a visitation from an angel. **Significance**: Joseph did as he was told, thus fulfilling the prophecy that the Lord would call His Son out of Egypt.
Joseph Matthew 2:22–23 Type: warning/direction	Upon the return to Israel, Joseph heard that Archelaus was reigning in Judea in Herod's place and he became afraid, so he was warned in a dream to go to Galilee to the town of Nazareth.	**Interpretation**: This dream could have been literal or it could have been symbolic and all that was recorded in the Bible was the interpretation. **Significance**: Following the dream, Joseph took the family to Nazareth, and so, the prophecy was fulfilled that the Savior would be called a Nazarene.
Pilate's Wife Matthew 27:19 Type: warning	While Pilate was sitting on the judge's seat, his wife sent him the message not to have anything to do with the innocent man (Jesus), because she had suffered a great deal that day in a dream because of Him.	**Interpretation**: This dream could have been literal or it could have been symbolic and all that was recorded in the Bible was the interpretation. **Significance**: When Pilate saw that he was getting nowhere with the chief priests and the elders concerning the innocent man, he took water and

Dreams Revealed:
Handbook for Biblical Dream Interpretation

Dream Info	Actual Dream	Interpretation and Significance
		washed his hands in front of the crowd, claiming that he was innocent of Jesus' blood and the responsibility of His death fell on the people.

UNIT 2:
WHAT TO DO WITH DREAMS

According to the Book of Joel, dreams, visions, and prophecies will increase in the last days and keep increasing until His coming.[28] It seems everyone will be dreaming or having visions. We need to make ourselves ready to understand the God-given messages in our dreams for ourselves and others.

WHAT NOT TO DO WITH YOUR DREAMS

Before diving in to what to do with dreams, it would behoove us to mention what NOT to do with dreams.

First of all, do NOT think that dream interpretation isn't biblical. The Bible is loaded with instances of God speaking to people through dreams, and how dreams in biblical times were held with extremely high regard. So why don't Christians still share this sentiment? The New Age movement is a spiritual movement that developed during the 1970s with the dawning of the Age of Aquarius and a free-spirit movement of non-conformity to social norms. New Age philosophies basically believe in a higher consciousness and self-awareness, as opposed to God. When Christians rejected the belief in dreams from God and discarded it, they just picked it up. (Sometimes our Christian attitudes and resistance toward the supernatural prevent us from moving in the fullness of blessings.)

Second, do NOT ignore dreams. If the Lord is trying to tell you something and you continually disregard Him, He may choose to stop. (And it is a grievous thing when the Lord stops talking.) In addition, repeatedly ignoring the messages, by not writing them down or thinking about them, will decrease your recall ability.

At first, I ignored my dreams, assuming they had little value. However, when I realized that God was talking to me, I had to have answers! Not only did I begin paying attention to my dreams, but I also embarked on my quest for a deeper understanding of dream interpretation.

Some dreamers think that if they are not receiving a Moses experience on the mountaintop and wake up with the equivalent of the Ten Commandments, it isn't God. Not all dreams are from God and not all dreams are meant to be remembered, but we should always be prepared nevertheless. When a dream seems minor and relatively insignificant, it hardly seems worth the effort. Looking back, there were hundreds of dreams I shelved thinking they were nonsense, and yet now, they make perfect sense. They either came to pass over time, or as I increased in understanding, the meanings became clear. If you do not understand your dream, write it down anyway. You are demonstrating the importance of dreams to God when you value what He gives you. Besides, if the Lord can trust us with small things (like a dream only thirty seconds long), then He will trust us with bigger things (like a whole night of dreaming). Just imagine how much He could tell us in that length of time!

Third, do NOT mishandle your dreams. Some dreamers misinterpret the message, thinking that the dream was about another person and then advise (or correct) that person based on what they thought God was showing them. Likewise, dreams should never be exaggerated or added to.

Finally, do NOT allow pride to find its way into your heart concerning dreams and God speaking to you. It is a privilege to receive revelation, but it is never sent to elevate us above others. Also, maintain a teachable spirit. There will be times when your interpretation of a dream is incorrect. Be open to skilled interpreters whom God may place in your life.

PRAY FOR YOUR DREAMS

Before you go to sleep each night, pray to receive dreams from God. If you have a specific need, pray for a dream to provide information and revelation to help you. Also, pray that you will remember the dream and be able to recall it in detail.

We have an enemy of our soul who would like nothing more than to shut off all communication between us and God. He will do anything to stop us from reaching our destiny, and he does not stop his pursuit just because we are sleeping. Each night before sleep, pray for the Lord to restrain the enemy and prevent him from filling your dreams with lies, confusion, and fear.

When you do receive a dream, pray and thank God for it. The Bible tells us to always give thanks to God for everything.[29] Regardless of the source of the dream, give thanks and pray that revelation is gleaned from it. If it is a dark dream from the enemy, recognize the plan and avoid that trap.

Pray for understanding of your dream and do not be afraid to ask God why you received it. If you pray without belief, you will not get very far. When you ask what your dream means, believe for the answer. Thank Him for direction and warnings.

Pray for instructions about how to follow up on the dream. Pray and ask the Lord what He wants you to do with the dream and ask for supernatural discernment. If you still are struggling with the understanding of the dream or how to handle it, pray for confirmation and clarification. Ask God to continue speaking to you about the issue over the next few nights in subsequent dreams.

RECORD YOUR DREAMS

After witnessing the benefit of dreams and how they come to pass, my biggest regret is not writing them down, especially in the early years.

If you have been dreaming for any length of time, then you know how quickly dreams can fade. As proof, try to recall what you dreamed a month ago. A dream can be fleeting, elusive, and difficult to catch unless it is one of those permanently imprinted on our conscience. If we do not make an effort to capture our dreams, then most of them will be lost. Many times I have awakened with an amazing dream that I feel sure I will never forget but it is gone before I make it to the kitchen.

Keeping records of your dreams will refresh your memory and show recurring themes. You can keep your dreams alive by reviewing them. It is fascinating to look back and see how the Lord reveals relevant and important information right when we need it.

I used to lose a lot of sleep getting up in the middle of the night to journal my entire dream, so I developed another system. Now, as soon as I am awake enough to realize I was dreaming, I jot down the key points in a notebook I keep beside my bed, then go right back to sleep and dreaming. The next day, I look over my notes and use them to write a detailed version of the dream in my official dream journal.

If you have trouble functioning well enough in the early hours to write a narrative of your dream, try a different approach such as drawing or voice recording. Just keep it simple. If it becomes complicated or too time-consuming you probably will not follow through. Create a habit that you become comfortable with.

You may be surprised how much more is available to you when you develop a system for yourself. Whatever method you use to record your dreams, it will take time and practice to acquire a habit. Even if you do not enjoy writing, try sticking with it long enough to see the benefits. Once you maintain this habit, hopefully you will be more inclined to embrace it.

Key Components to Capture

Just like in a mystery, look for the five Ws: who, what, when, where, and why. Who were the main players? Were you active in the dream or did it seem like you were mostly observing? Make a list to address the five Ws. Chances are—if you only capture this information, it will be enough to jog your memory about the dream the next day.

If you have the ability to capture more about the dream, begin jotting down additional aspects. Concentrate first on the things that really stick out or may have seemed out of place or character. Include any colors you noticed in the dream. Also, note any feelings you had during it. If you happen to notice the time you awake from the dream, make a note of it, too, because God could be giving you additional revelation about the dream. For example, the time may be referencing a Bible verse, a time of day, or a date.

Methods for Quick Capture

Dreams can be captured during the night via handwriting/drawing in a bedside notebook, typing on an electronic device, or voice recording. Following is a brief summary of the most popular techniques.

Scribbling the key points in a bedside notebook is probably the most used method. Even if you capture a single word, it can be enough to jolt your memory the next day. Not long ago, I scribbled the word *ahazrus*. It took several attempts to figure out the word, but eventually it dawned on me that I dreamed of King Ahasuerus (also known as Xerxes), whose wife, Esther, exposed an evil plot to kill the Jews in Persia. I knew the dream was a call for me to pray, "Dear Father, please raise up Your Esthers in the land to speak truth into leaders' ears and rescue Your people."

We all know that a picture is worth a thousand words. Sometimes a simple picture can quickly explain a dream better than lengthy text. You do not have to be an artist, because stick figures and elementary drawings will do fine. I tend to use drawings for things hard to explain, such as strange-looking items, scenery, or placement of people. You may wish to add a few words describing the drawing.

Diagramming, which can be traced back to Aristotle, is another quick-capture technique for dreams. The two main diagramming models are the cluster and linear ones (see Figure 2 for examples). The linear diagram uses straight lines and is more of a left brain activity, whereas the cluster diagram classifies and organizes information around related clusters and is more of a whole brain exercise, incorporating right and left brain thinking.

When I was in school, we used cluster diagrams for brainstorming and pre-writing exercises because it was free flowing and helped link ideas together. A modified version of cluster diagramming for use with dreams was coined by John Paul Jackson and is now used widely by many dreamers. Once you get the hang of his method, you can diagram a dream in just a few minutes.

Figure 2. Examples of Capturing a Dream with Diagramming

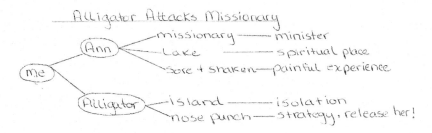

A stenographer's pad is a great tool for capturing the highlights of a dream (see Figure 3). The goal is to take notes on the left side of the line so that the next day, you can use the right side to add details or insert symbolic meanings to get a jump start on the interpretation. The downfall of using these pads is that you may feel like you are squishing information on the left if the dream is a long one with lots of details. This method will make more sense once you learn the basic dream interpretation techniques in Unit 3.

Figure 3. Example of Capturing a Dream with a Steno Pad

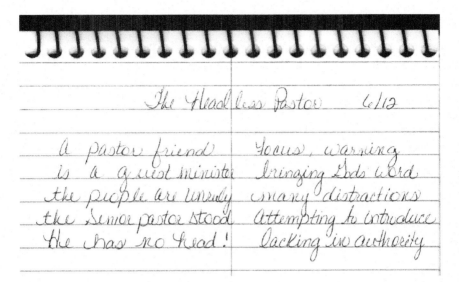

The Headless Pastor   6/12

A pastor friend   Focus, warning
is a guest minister   bringing Gods Word
the people are unruly   many distractions
the Senior pastor stood   Attempting to introduce
He has no head!   lacking in authority

Probably the easiest way to capture a dream in the middle of the night is via voice recording. Although there are lots of options out there for recording devices, the most logical one would be a cell phone. The biggest advantage of a cell phone is the ability to save a voice recording of a narration of the dream or to voice-text/e-mail it so that you don't have to write or type it the next day. The technology of voice-to-text has greatly improved the mission of capturing dreams without having to get out of bed.

Regardless of how you capture your dreams during the night, the following general tips will help you.

1) When you first awaken, take a minute to think about and remember your dream. Keep your mind quiet from competing thoughts. Even if you have no dream recollection, don't give up too fast. Allow the chance for your dream to be revealed.

2) Do not procrastinate once you remember the dream. It is difficult to rationalize the need to capture the dream when you are still half asleep. In the past, I would lie awake wrestling with the desire to go back to sleep, but concerned that if I did, the dream would be forgotten. Sometimes I would lie there twenty minutes thinking about it when it would have only taken a minute to jot it down.

3) Some people prefer using their tablets. If you do, dim your screen settings to reduce the light in your eyes, which may wake you too much and prevent you from returning to sleep.

Dream Journal

It is NOT enough to keep only the notes you captured during the night as your long-term collection of dreams. It is imperative that you use the notes to create a detailed description of the dream. You need to have an official dream journal.

> And the LORD answered me, and said, "Write the vision, and make it plain upon tables, that he may run that readeth it." (Habakkuk 2:2 KJV)

When I began my dream journey, I had no idea I would have so many dreams. I wrote them on anything I could find (including the back of junk mail and scrap paper). In other words, I could see the short-term value of dreams but not the long-term. You might as well accept the fact that you are wired to be a dreamer, and you are going to have many more dreams that need a special place. Just think: *if* you recall one dream a night, then that is 365 dreams per year or 3,650 dreams in ten years. You need a journal.

Your first decision is whether you will have an electronic journal, a handwritten journal, or a combination of both. My personal journal has a mixture of techniques that best fit each dream. There are cluster diagrams, simple drawings, summaries, lists, and old-fashioned written-out details. When I type out my dream, I usually save it to my computer, then print a copy so that I can write notes all over it and later place it in a folder (depending on the dream). If you type out your dream, then make a printed copy to use for writing; you can underline symbols, circle key words, and write notes in the margin to prepare it for the interpretation. At the bottom, I usually write my thoughts on the dream. You can also add applicable events going on in your life. Once you get an idea of the dream's meaning, you can go back and either write or type it in. This is important later when you see how the dream manifested in real life. You will see how close you were or where you missed the mark. Whatever you choose, be consistent at capturing your dreams.

For some dreams, you will want to remember every detail and give them your full attention. Be sure to write in a way you will understand rather than writing so others can follow it. The journal is for you. You can abbreviate, use nicknames, or whatever personalizes it for you.

Cluster diagrams are good for capturing the dream highlights, as well as the final detailed dream. Ask yourself whom the dream is mostly about, what it centers around, and where you are in the dream. Write the main subject of the dream in the center of your diagram. (The majority of your dreams will be about you.) If it is about you, you can simply write "me." Begin to expand the diagram with the most important details closest to the center, and the less weighty ones on the outer perimeters. Note: Nouns and pronouns tend to be toward the center while adjectives end up in the details.

Once you practice diagramming and get the hang of it, you may choose to journal your dreams using this method. Of course, writing out the whole dream will be more memorable, but when the dream is long, this is a good way to get it down quickly. The downside of using only a cluster in your journal is that the details seem to fade from your memory over time. For this reason, I would write an additional line or two summarizing the dream. More information about using cluster diagrams for interpretation is presented in Unit 3.

Regardless of how you format your dream journal, the following general tips will help you.

1) Writing/recording the dream in present tense makes it stay current and active. Use present-tense verbs such as: "I am" versus. "I was"; "she is" versus "she was"; "we are" versus "we were"; and "they are" versus "they were". Past-tense verbs create a sense that the message of the dream is in the past.

2) Be sure to add the date and time of your dream. Not only can this information pinpoint seasons in your life, they can be clues for scriptures or when the message of the dream may be needed in real life. For example, I once dreamed (on the third) that I checked into hotel room #3. The date of the dream was a confirmation that God was with me in a temporary situation (the hotel) that I was involved in at the time.

3) Add a title to every dream. It should be something catchy that relates to the dream, like a movie title. This will help you locate the dream later. Looking for a dream without a title is like looking for a needle in haystack.

4) Keep your journal private. Your journal is a private matter between you and God. The information can easily be misunderstood when others read it as if it were literal. One time, a woman shared with me that her husband was angry because she was dreaming about her ex-husband, even though she insisted that she did not have feelings for him. Unfortunately, her husband did not understand the symbolic nature of dreams, and that her dream did not have anything to do with her desire to reconcile with her ex; it was more about rejection and old wounds surfacing from that hurtful relationship.

5) Review your journal on a regular basis. Reviewing it often will help you connect dreams that are related and give you a better overview of what your dreams are telling you. Most dreams are time-sensitive and can be tied to past dreams. In other words, you may dream of something in multiple ways until you "get it." When you look over a series of dreams, you may notice that certain dream themes recur during certain seasons of your life. For example, during times of high stress, financial shifts, or transitional changes, you may regularly have dreams to help you resolve issues on the job (especially if you are about to make a wrong decision). You may also notice things beginning to smooth out, as the dreams decrease and switch to another theme.

6) Don't get frustrated if you cannot recall a dream or figure out what it means. We know from scripture that sometimes our instructions are sealed (see Job 33:16). Even with your best efforts, some dreams will be inaccessible because they are deposited into your spirit and bypass your mind. If you don't completely recall the dream, write the thoughts you were thinking upon waking. Sometimes it may take years to get the revelation of a dream because it may be for a later appointed time.

GET AN INTERPRETATION OF YOUR DREAMS

If God goes though the effort to give us a dream, then surely He expects us to seek an understanding of it. Learn to interpret your dreams!

Like any skill, the ability to interpret dreams will improve with practice over time. A good measure of Bible knowledge and discernment speeds up the process. You can learn to interpret dreams if you will put in the time and discipline. Unit 3 is an instructional short course to jump-start your journey.

Often, the hardest dreams to interpret are our own. If you do not know how to interpret your dream or have trouble doing so, then enlist the help of trusted friends or ministry leaders.

When you do receive an interpretation of a dream, make sure to record it in your dream journal. Not only is it fun to compare the interpretation to the actual unfolding of the events in our life, but also it shows us where we nailed it or details we may have missed. For the dreams that had a few lingering details, we will be able to look back and say, "Oh, so that's what that detail meant."

FOLLOW UP
ON YOUR DREAMS

When God spoke directly to the people in the Bible through dreams or visions, they were accountable for the revelation given. The same is true for us. Literal dreams have greater accountability because the message is crystal clear. John Paul Jackson aptly named it the "Clarity Cost." The greater the clarity, the greater the cost. Remember Abimelech, who was told to return Sarah to Abraham or die. To ignore a warning in a dream could cost lives. We are accountable for the messages from God whether we like it or not. But that is not all—we are accountable for how we follow up on the dream, as well.

To correctly follow up on a dream, we must use spiritual discernment. Since God is spirit, we can understand spiritual things only by revelation through the Holy Spirit, who expresses the heart of God to us. Our natural knowledge is limited by things such as our environmental influences, educational background, church teachings, and perspectives developed over our lifetime. It is difficult to understand spiritual revelation given in dreams and visions with our carnal, natural thinking. In fact, the Bible says spiritual things seem foolish to the natural mind.

> But the natural man receiveth not the things of
> the Spirit of God: for they are foolishness unto
> him: neither can he know them, because they
> are spiritually discerned. (1 Corinthians 2:14
> KJV)

Most of the time, our dreams are a call to action, and we
need discernment about how to proceed. For example, we
must determine whether we are supposed to tell people the
dreams we had about them or whether we were given inside
information about their life so that we could anonymously
pray for them.

The first step to acting on a dream is prayer. We always
need to ask the Lord why He gave the dream. Was it to
intercede for someone? Was it a warning about something
that is about to happen? Was it to reveal hidden sin to
show us where we need cleansing and prayer? The most
common mistake I see is when a dreamer REACTS to a
dream before praying and getting an accurate
interpretation. We must act, not react.

After getting an interpretation of a dream through prayer
and discernment, the next two steps are to measure it
against the Word of God and to find how it fits into our life.

Generally when God speaks to us in dreams, He is
providing information about the here and now. Rarely do
dreams concern distant future events. Sometimes they do
speak of the past, but even then, they are addressing
current feelings about past situations. When trying to plug
a dream in to your life, ask yourself what is happening
around you that the dream could relate to. Look for events
coming up, areas you are struggling with, or situations in
your business or home life.

On rare occasions, God will send an answer for someone else through one of our dreams, especially if they asked us to pray for them concerning the issue. For example, I have a friend who entered a national beauty pageant and she asked me to pray for her. I agreed and after prayer, I dreamed she was in her evening gown on a stage, and when she bowed to the crowd, the crown of her head was bald. I understood the dream to mean that her baldness indicated the lack of a victory crown.

In another dream-related situation, God provided an answer that intersected both my prayers and those of another lady. For several months I kept dreaming about Tammy, a friend from high school. Each dream was little different, but basically, I was waving at her from a hilltop while she was in her workplace in the valley. Sometimes I would have fruit to offer and would wave for her to come get it. She would always say that she was working and couldn't come right then. In the last dream I had, I went down to get her. She said she needed to finish up and would come in a minute. I smiled and told her that I would see her soon. I hadn't seen Tammy in years, so each time I woke up I would wonder why I kept dreaming about her. One day, while I was getting ready to put an ad in the paper for a job opening in our office, I heard a small inner voice tell me to go to the grocery store right then. Despite my reluctance to go and no need to purchase anything there, I made my way to the store. Standing in the bakery, I felt a little silly until I ran into Tammy. It did not take long for the two of us to assemble the pieces: Her job was ending and I had an opening. Just like in my dreams, I had something to offer her, but now, she was free to come get it. One series of dreams answered two women's prayers.

God appoints some dreamers to speak into the lives of leadership, and therefore, it is important to briefly discuss the protocol for sharing dreams with them. If you are given specific revelation about a church, ministry, or other group, I strongly believe it is unwise to tell them about it unless the Lord has dealt with your heart and you have a release to do so. Sharing the dream before you have understanding of it could undoubtedly cause confusion and dissension. Furthermore, we are not called to be accusers, even if we do so with good intentions. (We already have an accuser of the brethren, and his name is Satan.[30])

Care is especially warranted for "church" dreams. It is highly likely that most of these dreams are intended to cause us to pray, fast, and intercede, instead of meddle. It may actually be burdensome to the leadership to hear all our dreams about how to fix the church. The last thing we want is to blast the people of our church, make them suspicious of each other, or create dissension in the leadership. If we want revelation, the Lord has to be able to trust us with it. Handling church dreams requires MUCH prayer and wisdom.

A serious word of caution about dreams: don't become suspicious, judgmental, or angry with brothers and sisters in Christ because of a dream. You can be cautious without judgment. Be aware that dreams are highly metaphoric. That means the person in your dream may represent someone else or a prototype of that person. Sometimes a dream will not bear witness with your spirit or your experience with the person. If someone has shown you nothing but friendship, kindness, and love, then question a dream that shows otherwise. I know of spouses who wake up angry because they dreamed the other was cheating.

Most of the time, that is not the dream's meaning, which is probably instead indicating that the dreamer may feel cheated of time together, or that the spouse may be given to other passions such as work or hobbies. The enemy will try to put a wedge between marriages and friendships that are Christ-centered and attempt to replace them with counterfeits that encourage alienation from Christ. The bottom line is to be guilty of nothing but love.

KEEP THE FAITH

As parents, we want to tell our children everything they need to know, but sometimes, they are not able (or willing) to hear it all at once. So, knowing they will run across certain situations in life, we tend to squeeze advice in where we can in hopes that they will draw from the wisdom when the time comes. In the same way, the Lord deposits things in our spirit we do not yet understand, in order to prepare us for future circumstances.

> *I have yet many things to say unto you, but ye cannot bear them now.* (John 16:12 KJV)

There will be some dreams you will not be able to process because it is out of timing. Just go with what you are given and be in peace about it.

When we begin to doubt that the Holy Spirit is speaking to us in dreams or when the enemy is trying to convince us that dreams are foolish, it is a good time for us to reflect on the many blessings received through our dreams. We must recall the dreams that helped us when we were desperate for answers and remember the times when the Lord led us in the right direction because of a dream.

Always remember there is an enemy who wants us to abandon our dreams, shut out the kingdom, and walk in darkness. But we also have a GREAT BIG GOD who has plans to prosper us and give us a hope and a future.[31] Ask yourself if you have anything to lose by choosing to embrace your dreams. Consider the consequences of shutting this door of revelation in your life. It can happen when we drop our guard.

Review your journal and see how dreams have impacted your life. When you want to give up on your dreams, just choose to keep the faith.

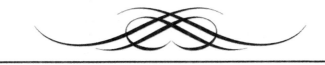

UNIT 3:
INTERPRETING DREAMS

This unit is designed to provide the how-tos for interpreting dreams. Please note that everything mentioned is based on biblical dream interpretation and ministry experience, as opposed to New Age methods.

DREAM LANGUAGE

One of the most perplexing concepts to grasp regarding dreams is the way God speaks. On one hand, we have the literal letter of the law and absolutes that are black and white, while on the other hand, we have metaphors and symbolism, which can be colorful, creative, and mysterious.

Like the Bible, our dreams are filled with figurative language and parables, both of which add a richer and deeper understanding of the message. Figurative language stretches us to think in unusual ways that divert our thinking from the logical and predictable, thus keeping us from becoming spiritually rigid. This form of revelation also keeps us from becoming self-righteous and proud of all that God is revealing. We cannot be very prideful when we spend most of our day walking around trying to figure out what God is saying to us.

Metaphors and Similes

A metaphor is a comparison between two typically unrelated things. It is a representation used to relate one thing to something else. There are plenty of examples of metaphors in the Bible. In Matthew 13:18–23, Jesus used soil as a metaphor to represent our hearts, seeds for the Word, and thorns and briars for the wicked.

The Holy Spirit and Jesus are described in metaphors to give us a glimpse of their power, glory, majesty, and holiness. Metaphors help paint a picture for us that is familiar and easy to relate to. Some metaphor examples for the Holy Spirit include breath,[32] living water,[33] and wind.[34] Some metaphor examples for Jesus include:

Cornerstone[35]	Bread of Life[36]	Bridegroom[37]
Fountain[38]	Forerunner[39]	Foundation[40]
Rock[41]	Gate[42]	Gift[43]
Beginning[44]	Lamb[45]	Word[46]
Life[47]	Lion of Judah[48]	Rising Sun[49]
Truth[50]	Stone[51]	The Amen[52]
Morning Star[53]	Vine[54]	Door[55]
The Way[56]	Resurrection[57]	Alpha and Omega[58]
Lily of the Valley[59]	Rose of Sharon[60]	Horn of Salvation[61]
Branch of the Lord[62]	Light of the World[63]	

A simile is a comparison between two things using words such as *like* or *as*. For example: The kingdom of heaven <u>is like</u>
* a merchant looking for fine pearls.[64]
* a man who sowed good seed in his field.[65]
* a mustard seed.[66]
* a treasure hidden in a field.[67]
* a net that was let down into the lake.[68]

A simile has more of an implied meaning, while a metaphor is direct. A metaphor states that something "IS," while a simile states that it "IS LIKE" or "AS."

Metaphor: The <u>lion</u> (enemy) <u>is</u> come up from his thicket, and the destroyer is on his way.[69]

Simile: He (the enemy) lies in wait secretly <u>like</u> <u>a lion</u> in his den.[70]

Parables

A parable is a short story that teaches a moral or spiritual lesson.[71] Jesus often taught in parables. When asked why, His response was:

> *"Because the knowledge of the secrets of the kingdom of heaven has been given to you, but not to them. Whoever has will be given more, and they will have an abundance. Whoever does not have, even what they have will be taken from them. This is why I speak to them in parables: Though seeing, they do not see; though hearing, they do not hear or understand."* (Matthew 13:11–13 NIV).

The Bible says that it is the glory of God to conceal a thing, but the honor of kings is to search it out.[72] Parables invite us into a story to dig for that treasure, as described in Matthew 13:44.

The greatest strength of parables is their ability to be remembered over long periods of time and to be applied to several different situations.

In general (and I state this without putting God in a box), when God needs to communicate something to us urgently and without the possibility of misunderstanding, He will tend to do so with more literal language as opposed to parables. On the other hand, when He needs for us to ruminate on ideas for a longer period of time, the information or revelation may come in parable form so that it is more easily remembered and digested. Symbolic dreams are nothing less than nighttime parables from the Lord.

Symbols

When I began my dream journey, people would say, "Just pray for the interpretation," and I agree with that, but there is something else you need to understand—*symbolism.*

Unit 4 is a comprehensive dream symbol dictionary to get you started. The symbols used in this dictionary are intended to help you build your dream vocabulary. The dictionary is NOT meant to give the impression that dream interpretation is a formulaic process whereby a person can substitute definitions from the dictionary into their dreams and get a message from God. Instead, it is a tool to open understanding of symbolic language and discussions with the Holy Spirit.

It is important to note that there are positive and negative meanings for just about every symbol. Consider the context to determine which direction the symbol is pointing. For example, a red apple in a positive connotation could represent something you love that is healthy for you (red = love; apple = healthy, as in "an apple a day keeps the doctor away"). In a negative connotation, the red apple could represent something that looks sweet on the outside but is toxic if you sink your teeth into it (many cartoon princesses can attest to this).

In itself, the dictionary in Unit 4 is in no way complete because, as you can see, there are infinite possible meanings for any single symbol, all depending on the context in which it is used. What location is to real estate, context is to symbolism—it makes all the difference. As you grow in your dream interpretation experience and your dream vocabulary expands, continue to add your own symbols and meanings to the dictionary.

Animals

Many animals have physical characteristics that distinguish them from others. For example, a raccoon appears to be wearing a bandit mask, a vulture is bald, and a giraffe is a head above the rest. In addition, all animals have behaviors that set them apart. For example, a boa constrictor squeezes the life out of its prey, a peacock has a prideful demeanor, and a hyena appears to laugh. Some animals are concentrated in certain geographical areas or perhaps are mascots for a group, and therefore, are associated with those places. For example, the panda could symbolize China, a bear could symbolize Russia, or a cardinal could represent either a baseball team or St. Louis.

Animals are associated with advertisements, store logos, products, and cultural icons too. Several years ago, I was asked by a social worker to help a teen resolve some issues in her home life. The night before our meeting, I dreamed the teen sat motionless and expressionless looking out of a large window. In the adjoining window was a basset hound in the same stance. When I awoke, I realized that the dog looked vaguely familiar. Then it dawned on me, it was the logo for Hush Puppies shoes. The dream indicated that the teen would not open up at our meeting, and sure enough, she didn't. She was one "hushed" puppy.

Animals can represent a variety of situations in the *dreamer's* life. For example, a pit bull to an extreme dog lover may mean one thing, but to a victim of a pit-bull attack, it could be something totally different. The situation in the *animal's* life can provide clues, too. Consider the appropriate habitat for the animal and see whether the dream locale fits. Perhaps the dream is about a fish out of water or a dolphin in a bird's nest. Consider the implications of these sorts of mismatches.

More times than not, animals in our dreams represent people we know, like a weasel could be someone trying to back out of an obligation. A man in our dream class dreamed a polar bear was chasing him. The dream was a warning that a coldhearted, religious spirit would try to attack him. A few days later, someone verbally attacked him because he was a Christian.

A quick Internet search may be necessary if you are not familiar with the animal. You do not need to know everything about it, just the main characteristics. Consider special markings, color, and behavior patterns. Look for wordplays such as: "gorilla/guerilla warfare," "loan shark," "pet issue," or "skunked."

Ask why you dreamed of that particular animal and whether it was good or bad. A dog protecting you could mean a friend is standing in the gap offering protection for you, but a dog that turns on you and bites your backside is a warning to watch for backbiters. Watch out for contradictions, too. Not all animals that are white (usually symbolizing cleanness and holiness) are good. An example is a white rat that could represent something in your life appearing clean on the outside, but is really drawn to filth. If the animal is a pet in the dream, but not in reality, consider the possibility that you may have a pet issue that needs be addressed. As always, consider the context of the dream.

Colors

Colors in scripture have specific significance according to their use and value. For example, blue dye (*tekheleth*, taken from a shellfish) was applied to the tassels of a four-cornered garment, the veil of Solomon's Temple, vestments, embroideries, tapestries of the tabernacle, and adornments for the palace. Blue was used for royal and priestly garments and furnishings.[73] Purple was highly prized and rare due to the difficulty in finding and extracting the dye from a small gland found in the neck of the mollusk and other Mediterranean shellfish. Purple was associated with wealth and nobility and was also used for royal apparel and furnishings.[74]

In the color palette, hue is the name given to a color (i.e., red, yellow, green, orange). Intensity is the strength or vividness of the color, and value is the lightness or darkness of the color.

Red, yellow, and blue cannot be achieved by mixing other colors to create them, and thus are referred to as primary colors. Secondary colors are a mixture of two primary colors. A dream that is in all primary colors could be talking about something that is or needs to be primary in our life.

Pastels can indicate a softer or immature version and suggest that something is still developing into its fullness. For example, green symbolizes life, and therefore, someone wearing a pastel green shirt could represent a person who is young, inexperienced (a new employee is called "green"), or not fully mature in an area of life. Bright colors are designed to grab our attention and imprint something into our memory.

Color is one of the most important details in a dream, especially if the dream has only a few memorable ones. Consider how informative the colors are in the following examples. A bright blue coat could be a covering or call to revelation and communion with God. A green hat could be someone's conscience bothering him. Red shoes could indicate someone is walking in wisdom, power, and anointing. Sometimes a color is not "pure" so to speak, and is a mixture of two other colors. Turquoise is a mixture of blue, green, and white; teal is blue and green, and pink is red and white. For colors you are unsure about, you can symbolically define them by the composite colors, all while keeping the dreamer and context in mind. A rainbow to some people may represent God's promises, but to others, it could symbolize gay and lesbian rights.

The Word of God says that God is light and in Him there is no darkness.[75] Every existing color is part of pure white light and can be seen when a prism separates it. On the contrary, black is not considered a color; it is the absence of light, and therefore, color.

Most dream leaders agree that black-and-white dreams are likely from the enemy or the soul, and mostly dark and black dreams are definitely from the enemy. However, caution is certainly warranted. While God can give us whatever kind of dream He wants, He generally reserves His all–black-and-white dreams for topics dealing with discernment and for which there is no room for gray areas.

Just like with other symbols, colors are used as part of wordplays and idioms. In our dream class, a man said he dreamed about a big blue figure following him. When one of our team members asked if he struggled with depression ("the blues"), he admitted that it had been a problem following him throughout his life. Other expressions involving color include blackballed (excluded, ostracized, socially rejected), greenhorn (inexperienced), yellow-bellied (cowardly), and red-handed (caught doing something wrong).

Look for colors in your dream that seem out of ordinary. A friend shared a dream in which a pink key appeared over her head. The image symbolized the ability to unlock things for women. The Lord was affirming her ministry with women and confirming that He had given her the key to unlock destiny, callings, and potential in their lives.

Dreams may be colorful, muted, or neutral. There may be a single color that stands out or something that seems illuminated. When contemplating a color in a dream, be sure to consider all the qualities it possesses.

Numbers

The Bible has a lot to say about numbers—so much so that there is even an entire book in the Old Testament called *Numbers*.

Numbers are important to God. He knows the exact number of hairs on your head[76] and stars in the heavens.[77] And have you read the detailed measurements for the temple and tabernacle? Our God pays incredible attention to detail. When the words *count, measure,* or *weight* are used in the Bible, it is specific and purposeful. This is not numerology, but is God's divine order. There are deeper meanings implied than the simple number itself. Consider the number seven, which symbolizes fulfillment, completion, and accomplished works.

* The priests sprinkled blood and oil <u>seven</u> times each on the <u>seven</u> pieces of furniture in the tabernacle.

* The Israelites marched around Jericho for <u>seven</u> days and <u>seven</u> times on the <u>seventh</u> day.

* Hebrew slaves are to be set free in the <u>seventh</u> year, and the land is to rest every <u>seven</u> years.

* There are <u>seven</u> colors in a rainbow, <u>seven</u> days in a week, and <u>seven</u> annual Holy Days. The <u>seventh</u> day of the week is the Sabbath Day.

* God's Word is pure, like silver purified <u>seven</u> times in the fire.

* In the Book of Revelation, there are <u>seven</u> letters written to the <u>seven</u> churches, <u>seven</u> stars in Jesus' right hand representing the <u>seven</u> angels of the <u>seven</u> churches, <u>seven</u> golden lampstands representing the <u>seven</u> spirits of God, <u>seven</u> seals, <u>seven</u> trumpets, and <u>seven</u> bowls of wrath.

The number twelve (which symbolizes divine government and order) is also prevalent in scripture.

* There were <u>twelve</u> judges in Israel and <u>twelve</u> disciples.

* There are <u>twelve</u> stones in the breastplate representing the <u>twelve</u> tribes of Israel.

* Joshua called <u>twelve</u> men from the <u>twelve</u> tribes to shoulder <u>twelve</u> stones from the middle of the Jordan.

* There are <u>twelve</u> months in a year and <u>twelve</u> members on a court jury.

* A remnant of 144,000 (<u>twelve</u> x <u>twelve</u> x 1000) people will be sealed and stand with Jesus on Mount Zion before the final battle.

* The church bride wears a crown with <u>twelve</u> stars.

* The New Jerusalem has <u>twelve</u> gates with <u>twelve</u> angels at the gates with the names of the <u>twelve</u> tribes inscribed on them.

Number meanings can be literal or symbolic. If a number stands out in a dream, it is usually there for a reason. If a number does not seem important, jot it down in your dream journal just in case, and move on to other symbols.

People

Our brains naturally want to process symbols literally instead of symbolically. Discerning people in our dreams is probably the hardest of all, because they can be a mixture of literal and symbolic. In other words, one person in the dream may be that literal person, while another may be symbolic of something else. For example, I ministered to a married couple in which the man dreamed his wife was leaving him. He became suspicious of her and regularly reminded her of his dream, thus causing an emotional drain on their relationship. She shared that she never had thoughts of leaving him and admitted that she had become busy with a consuming project at work. The husband's feelings of abandonment and insecurity were causing him to dream about his wife's adulterous relationship; however, the person she was cheating with was not literal—it was symbolic for her work. As you can see, people in our dreams can be difficult to categorize, especially when strong feelings are attached to them.

When trying to ascertain the people in your dream, ask yourself first what your association with them is. Is the person a coworker, part of a particular church group, a family member, or a friend? Determine in which circle in your life they exist so that you can know whether the dream is speaking about your work, school, home, personal life, etc.

Other questions to ask concerning people in dreams include what is their main attribute or character, or what is their role or responsibility in life. For example, if you dream of the president showing up at your work, it could represent something political going on. A CEO or boss often represents the Lord (as one having authority). A judge in a dream may represent God or someone else who has the ability to decide fate in the dreamer's life, especially when justice is needed in a situation.

Strangers in dreams are often easier to evaluate because there is no emotional tie to the dreamer to muddy the interpretation. Faceless people in dreams can be spirits, angels, or the Holy Spirit. The actions of the stranger are key to its symbolism. Questions to answer include whether they were positive or negative, helpful or hurtful, and safe or scary. If the stranger has a name, the name itself could be a symbol. If the name is Gabriel, it could indicate angelic protection. If it is Elijah, there could be a prophetic message that the Lord is trying to send. Research the name for its meaning.

Unless urgent intercession is required and the Lord can trust you with it, rarely do we have dreams about other people's personal secrets or sins. Before we bring correction to others because of what we dreamed, we should first consider that the dream probably is about us. Although it may seem our dream is about the people we see in it, most dreams are really about our own issues.

Places

When we dream of a building or a particular place, it is often a situation or the condition dealing with an area of our life. It can involve home, family, job, health, ministry, work, or future places we will walk in. The type of building or its intended function will provide the context. For example, if the dream occurs in a gym, then we may need to work something out; if in a hospital, then we may need healing or restoration; if in an airport terminal, then we may be in a transition waiting to go higher. A dream with a building from our past (like a childhood home) could be addressing issues from our past. The condition of the building or place will provide context concerning what it looks like from a spiritual perspective (i.e., disrepair, confusion, annihilated, new, or refurbished/reclaimed). Buildings can be people, too: a bank could be the person who gives us our allowance or signs our paycheck.

If the dream occurs in a building, the precise room may be important. In a house, the family room (which is a casual place where family gathers) may speak of personal family issues; the kitchen is the heart of the home and the place of preparation of nourishment; a bedroom is a place involving rest or intimacy; and a bathroom is where we get relief from pressures building up inside us.

Transportation and Means of Movement

In general, when you think of transportation, think of something you are operating in or doing in your life, ministry, or occupation—basically, what drives you. It may also be a group or association involvement, especially if other people are on board or riding with you.

The size and function of the vehicle is important when it comes to our capacity to influence or carry others. Consider a dream occurring on a ship. If we are on a large ship with people from our church, we could be part of a movement in a mission-minded church. It does not necessarily mean we are physically going overseas, although we may. If the ship carries people from our workplace, then it could represent our sphere of influence to reach others with a product or service. As another example, a small plane is usually a small business, organization, or personal ministry. Therefore, a large jet could represent a large corporation or ministry with the potential for national or international influence (one that could move rapidly at a high level).

The reason and circumstances of transportation are informative, as is the condition of the vehicle. For example, is it reckless, too fast, too slow, or going in reverse? Does the dreamer end up in good places or bad ones? A dream about a car running on empty may be a warning that we need to refuel by getting back in the Word of God.

Our companions during the travel experience can provide context, too. Consider who is driving (and thus in control), who is just along for the ride, and who is taking a backseat. Where is the dreamer amongst the other people?

Like with animals and buildings, various vehicles can represent people. Consider the type of people who would be represented by a Hummer, a Corvette, or a tractor-trailer truck.

Context

No doubt, you have figured out by now that the key to symbolism is context. One single symbol can have a hundred different meanings in a hundred different dreams. This is why the Holy Spirit is absolutely necessary in biblical dream interpretation, because without Him, it is impossible to choose the correct meaning for the symbol.

As an illustration of the importance of context, the "if this, not that" technique is very helpful. Consider the following dream and the implications of changing a single symbol. For this demonstration, the meaning of the symbol is placed in brackets.

> *You dream that you are driving* [you are in control] *a red* [wisdom] *Infiniti car* [ministry of eternal purposes] *in the state of Arizona* [state motto is God enriches].

The message could be that you have a ministry to passionately enrich the lives of others and prepare them for their eternal purpose.

BUT—What if a thief and not you were driving? The message would change to indicate that the enemy has somehow gained control of your ministry and is driving it, and you need to get it back.

BUT—What if the car was a taxi and not an Infiniti? The message would change to indicate that you have a ministry to get people to where they need to be, thereby enriching their life.

BUT—What if you were parked and not driving? The message would change to indicate that you are stalled in your ministry and getting nowhere.

Context is everything.

Steps to Interpret a Dream

Of course, the first step of dream interpretation is prayer, but because this should be automatic, it is not considered an official step in the process.

Following is a three-step basic process for interpreting a dream. It is important to note, though, that the process actually involves more than three simple steps; however, these guidelines will help get you started on the path to understanding your dreams.

1. Identify the Focus, Subfocus, and Important Details.

The terminology *focus* and *subfocus* were first coined as part of dream interpretation by John Paul Jackson, who is considered in many circles to be a founding father of biblical dream interpretation.

Focus

The focus is the person or thing the dream is about. Finding the focus of the dream is top priority. We must know who the dream is about in order to apply the interpretation correctly.

To help determine what the focus is, use the following questions.

* Are you active or an observer in the dream?

* What is the one thing in the dream that, if removed, would cause the entire dream to not work?

* Who you are talking about the most when you tell the dream?

* Are you in most of the scenes?

If you are participating in the dream and involved in the main plot, then you are probably the focus. Most dreams we have are about ourselves. (Prayer intercessors have more dreams about other people as compared with non-intercessors.) God enjoys speaking to His children. If He wants to speak to our neighbor, He will most likely speak through their dreams and not ours. Since most dreams have something to do with the dreamer, look there first. More often than not, the dream is about the dreamer.

If you are only observing in a dream, the focus could be what or whom you are observing. Consider the following dream: *I am watching the tree blow back and forth in the wind. The green leaves are blowing away.* The dreamer is observing, and therefore, the focus is the tree.

Often messages sent in dreams are warnings, current issues or events in our lives either now or upcoming. It is vitally important that we understand who the dream is about. Missing the focus of the dream could cause us to misinterpret the dream.

Subfocus

The subfocus is who or what surrounds and supports the focus of the dream, and there can be more than one in each dream. The wind and leaves are subfocuses in the dream about the tree blowing back and forth. If we take these items out of the dream, the meaning would change because key elements are missing. To tell the difference between the tree (focus) versus the wind and leaves (subfocuses)—if we remove the tree from the dream, we would have no dream, while if we remove the wind or leaves, we only lose key pieces to the dream.

Important Details

Important details are helpful for building the foundation for the dream. In the dream about the swaying tree, the color green is an important detail because it tells us that the tree is losing live leaves instead of the expected dead ones. Try to avoid the common mistake of getting caught up in the details.

Using a Cluster Diagram

A cluster diagram is helpful for compartmentalizing the elements of a dream in order of importance.

Place the focus of the dream in the center of the page because it is what everything else centers around. Draw three lines (preferably no more to keep the diagram simple) radially out from the focus (like spokes on a wheel) and write the subfocuses at the end of each one. To each subfocus add a couple of details that support it. If there are some important details that go along with the focus, add those, too. See Figure 4 for a cluster diagram.

If you have a long dream with multiple scenes, you can make a separate diagram for each scene. When you get to the interpretation part, you will interpret each diagram separately and combine the overall meaning at the end.

Alternatively, you can treat the theme of each scene as a subfocus and create a single diagram. However, it is easier to interpret several smaller sections at a time and tie them together at the end, especially for beginners.

2. Define Symbols.

For each item on your diagram, choose a couple of symbolic meanings from the dream dictionary that may apply and add them beside the element (see Figure 4). Try to choose both a positive and negative meaning unless you are certain which to use. With multiple meanings in the symbol dictionary, you will need to consider the context of the dream to see which definition fits. If you feel none of them apply, do a little research. If it is a wordplay, you may check an online idiom dictionary, search the scriptures, use a standard dictionary, and do an Internet search for Christian-based resources.

Figure 4. Example of a Cluster Diagram

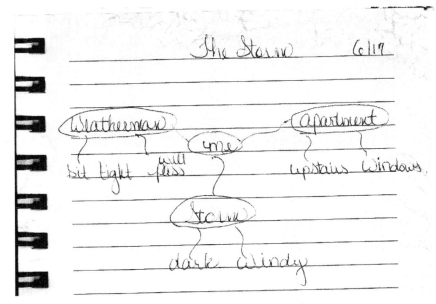

If you are using a narrative-based method for interpretation instead of a cluster diagram, somehow denote the focus, subfocuses, and details and add the possible symbolic meanings beside each one. Alternatively, you can make a separate list of the elements and place the symbolic meanings beside them.

Symbols are useful tools to help us with symbolic meanings, but discernment from the Holy Spirit is our guide through the process. When we sense something is right and apply it to the dream in a way that works, we are discerning and will feel a peace about it.

3. Form an Interpretation.

Knowing how to put the dream together requires skill, practice, and above all, the Holy Spirit. Sometimes we can piece the dream together like a puzzle and other times the pieces do not seem to fit well. A symbol in itself is just a piece of the dream and will not yield a whole interpretation. Don't be afraid to venture outside of the dream dictionary and think outside the box.

What type of dream is it? (For a review, see Unit 1.) This information will tell us which direction to go for the interpretation. For example, a dreamer swimming in water could mean they are moving in the Holy Spirit, and we would lean toward an optimistic interpretation. However, if the dreamer is struggling or drowning, the dream could be a warning about being overwhelmed, and thus we would lean toward a warning type of interpretation.

Reduce the dream to the essentials and connect the symbolic meanings of the dream. Pay attention to unusual things in the dream and conflicts. Create a brief synopsis that captures the overall essence and message. To get started, try to retell the dream in three sentences or less while using the symbolic meanings of the dream instead of the symbols themselves. Revise your interpretation as needed. If you are getting confused, check to see if you are overanalyzing it or fixating on certain details.

Once you have a basic interpretation, verify that it lines up with the Word of God. For example, it is not God's nature to cause us to judge others, retaliate, isolate ourselves, commit adultery, or have pride or any form of unforgiveness. If an interpretation suggests that we should embrace any of these sins, it is not congruent with the Word.

Before finalizing the interpretation, make sure that it is objective, especially if the dream does not belong to you.

Being objective means being open and also moving our own expectations out of the way. We all have our own perception of reality based upon our experiences and culture, whether it is real or not. Even when we get divine revelation or strategies in a dream, it can be clouded with confusion due to a lack of openness to alternative outcomes. Whether we admit it or not, our own desires can muddy situations, especially after we have prayed and waited for them. We must check into our mind and rake out all thoughts, ideas, and expectations to make a clearing for possibilities other than our own reasoning. Years ago, I dreamed that I stood gazing into a crystal-clear pond encircled by white flowers. Suddenly, my mother rose straight up out of the water in a white robe with her eyes fixed toward heaven. She took three steps toward the bank then ascended into the clouds. Despite my calls to her, she didn't seem to hear because she was captivated by something I couldn't see. When I awoke, I rejected any notion that her time was drawing near. Nevertheless, about a year later, tests revealed that she had cancer, and within three weeks she passed away. My objectivity had clouded the interpretation of the dream, and I failed to see God's prophetic warning.

When interpreting dreams for others, extra objectivity and care are needed. We should be careful to speak honestly, without embellishment or exaggeration, when reporting a dream. We should not go beyond what the dream is saying or say what is not there, either because we desire a certain outcome or wish to manipulate others with our information. We must keep our opinions in check. The best approach is to hit the highlights of the interpretation and let the Holy Spirit work on the rest with the person. In addition, the interpretation should be seasoned with grace and line up with the prophetic requirements to edify, exhort, or comfort (see 1 Cor 14:3).

Sometimes we will have to give interpretations that will be difficult for dreamers to hear, particularly if the message addresses hidden sin in their life. If we give the interpretation in a harsh way, the dreamer may reject it along with the harshness, yet if the interpretation is too diluted, they may dismiss it as irrelevant. For example, if a woman dreamer is dealing with lust, we would not want to tell her that she has the heart of a harlot. Instead, we may say something like, "The dream shows that you are struggling in this area and healing is available for you." We should express to the dreamer why God gave the dream (i.e., "I believe God gives this dream to encourage you, warn you, prepare you, make you aware..."). If it is a warning dream, we need to look for a positive outcome if it exists, and if it does not, then issue a strong warning while still expressing God's love and concern for them. The Lord does not give dreams to condemn anyone, but to give hope, life, and a future.

INTERPRETATION EXAMPLES

Following are ten real-life dream examples you can use to practice dream interpretation. Read through each dream and consider the focus, subfocus, and details. Once you formulate your own interpretation, check it against the one provided. Also, for more interpretation practice, you can use the biblical dreams provided in (Table 1).

Example 1: Driving Without Brakes

I am driving my car and can't seem to find the brakes. When I do find them, they do not work. I am looking for a mechanic along the way.

Focus, *Subfocus*, *and Important Details*

I am driving my car and can't seem to find the brakes. When I do find them, they do not work. I am looking for a mechanic along the way.

Symbols

Car = the dreamer's work, ministry, or what "drives" him

Brakes = ability to control stopping or slowing

"Putting the brakes on" = an idiom

Mechanic = Jesus, who can fix the problem

(The interpretation is on the next page.)

Interpretation

This is a warning (and direction) dream showing that you are having trouble saying no or "putting the brakes on" in some area of your life. The Lord will help restore control when you submit to Him. This dream was given to make you aware the Lord has what you need to get control back in your life.

Example 2: My Grandparents' Jewelry Box

I am in my grandparents' house, in a room I used to play in with a jewelry box. The jewelry box used to contain costume jewelry, but it was cleaned out except for a large red ruby. I feel it is for me.

Focus, Subfocus, and Important Details

I am in my grandparents' house, in a room I used to play in with a jewelry box. The jewelry box used to contain costume jewelry, but it was cleaned out except for a large red ruby. I feel it is for me.

Symbols

Grandparents' house = generational

Ruby = valuable items, such as blessings or anointing

Red = wisdom

(The interpretation is on the next page.)

Interpretation

This is a calling dream showing a generational blessing of wisdom and anointing passed to you from your grandparents. As childish things are now behind you, there is an invitation to pick up something precious to carry in your life. The dream was given to show you the valuable blessing left as your spiritual inheritance.

Example 3: The Storm

I am in an upstairs apartment that has a lot of windows. It becomes dark, very windy, and stormy. I am thinking that I need to leave as the storm grows worse. Our local weatherman is standing on the ground outside, with a big umbrella, yelling the weather report. He says, "We are having a terrible storm, but sit tight. It will pass quickly."

Focus, *Subfocus,* and <u>*Important Details*</u>

I am in an <u>upstairs</u> apartment that has a lot of <u>windows</u>. It becomes <u>dark</u>, very <u>windy</u>, and stormy. I am thinking that I need to leave as the storm grows worse. Our local weatherman is standing on the ground outside, with a big umbrella, yelling the weather report. He says, "We are having a terrible storm, but sit tight. It will pass quickly."

Symbols

Storm = difficulty, anger, "raging"

Upstairs = a higher perspective

Apartment = a temporary place or home life

Windows = vision to see the spiritual atmosphere

Sudden darkness = from the enemy rather than the Lord

Wind = something stirring up things

Weatherman = a prophetic voice

"Weather the storm" = an idiom meaning to wait it out

(The interpretation is on the next page.)

Interpretation

This is a warning dream telling you to prepare for a stormy time approaching. This could come in the form of anger or someone stirring something up around your home life. You will be able to see from a higher perspective and take comfort in knowing that if you sit tight, it will quickly pass. The Lord gives this dream to prepare you and give strategy to "weather the storm."

Example 4: Giving Birth in a Church Classroom

I am pregnant and looking into church classrooms that appear to be little artsy shops. I decide to work in the floral designing room. While working, I realize that it is time to give birth. The master floral designer comes to my aid along with the artist from her classroom. They are like midwives, helping me to deliver the baby. The doctor comes in dressed in white, but I cannot see his face.

Focus, Subfocus, and Important Details

I am pregnant and looking into church classrooms that appear to be little artsy shops. I decide to work in the floral designing room. While working, I realize that it is time to give birth. The master floral designer comes to my aid along with the artist from her classroom. They are like midwives, helping me to deliver the baby. The doctor comes in dressed in white, but I cannot see his face.

Symbols

Midwives = those who help release new things

Baby = new development, project, or ministry

Giving birth = timing is now; push to get project or ministry out

Church classroom = spiritual place of learning, ministry, training, equipping, teaching

Pregnant = something new developing

Master floral designer = Holy Spirit; imparts creative, living gifts

Doctor = Jesus, the Healer and Deliverer

(The interpretation is on the next page.)

Interpretation

This calling dream, about mentoring and birthing a new creative program for the church that will bless others, shows that the Lord has been training and developing your gifts, and it is now time to use them for the Body of Christ. It is a beautiful, fragrant, and pleasant gift. The Lord will help you bring this forth and offer support and assistance in this new and potentially fragile, life-giving (spiritually) program.

Example 5: My Formal Son in a Fast-Food Restaurant

My son, dressed in formal attire, is in a fast-food restaurant. It is messy and greasy; some French fries are on the floor. He looks surprised that his order is expensive. There are a few others inside dressed formally, too, but most people are dressed casually.

Focus, *Subfocus*, and *Important Details*

My son, dressed in formal attire, is in a fast-food restaurant. It is messy and greasy; some French fries are on the floor. He looks surprised that his order is expensive. There are a few others inside dressed formally, too, but most people are dressed casually.

Symbols

Son = natural or spiritual son

Fast-food restaurant = a place of spiritual teaching or information that is modified to make it palatable, fast, and low-cost, but has depleted nutritional value; business or personal choices (who you are allowing to feed you)

Formal attire = elegance; style; social influence; something you are called to do and only a few around you are making similar choices

Expensive = costing more than it is worth; sense of loss

Casual = informal; requires little personal preparation

(The interpretation is on the next page.)

Interpretation

This is a warning dream about the choices your son (literal or spiritual) is making (or going to make), whereby quality is sacrificed for the sake of convenience. He is making choices that are substandard to what he is called and equipped for. The Lord gives this dream for you to offer prayer, support, and encouragement for your son to reach higher and not to settle for second best.

Example 6: Alligator Attacks Missionary

Some minister friends and I are on a pontoon boat anchored in the middle of a lake. As some of us are swimming, I see an alligator emerge. I escape and make it to the bank, but the alligator grabs Ann by her midsection and takes her to a little island in the lake. As I wonder what to do, a sense of boldness comes over me. I swim to the island and punch the gator in the nose until it releases her. She is sore and shaken, but okay.

Focus, *Subfocus*, and *Important Details*

Some <u>minister</u> friends and ☐I☐ are on a pontoon boat anchored in the middle of a <u>lake</u>. As some of us are swimming, I see an <u>alligator</u> emerge. I escape and make it to the bank, but the ⌐alligator⌐ grabs ⌐Ann⌐ by her midsection and takes her to a <u>little island</u> in the lake. As I wonder what to do, a sense of boldness comes over me. I swim to the island and <u>punch</u> the gator in the nose until it releases her. She is <u>sore and shaken, but okay</u>.

Symbols

Alligator = person with influence and a dangerous big mouth that bites (slanders) and a powerful tail/tale; will try to take you under

Ann = a missionary friend who is being victimized

Ministers = people who teach, minister, and shepherd

Lake = spiritual condition or place (church or group)

Small island = isolation

Punch = spiritual warfare/intercession; fighting for others

(The interpretation is on the next page.)

Interpretation

This is a warning dream about the enemy's plan to prey on a missionary's personal life by bringing a vicious verbal attack affecting the ministry she is involved in. A vicious accusation will surface, leaving the minister isolated and wounded, but intercession from you will bring a release and freedom. Although recovery time may be needed for healing, there will be restoration.

Interesting Follow-Up

I had not seen Ann in over a year because she lived far away, but due to the serious nature of the dream, I contacted her. She explained that accusations from a person in her church had wounded her so deeply that she chose to step down from her position. Someone spoke against her past personal life, based on a rumor they heard. She said some of it was true prior to her salvation when she was young, but it was presented in a twisted way. She also felt alone (isolated) and was still recovering. She was actually relieved about the dream because she said no one but God would understand what she was going through. Today, her ministry is thriving more than ever.

Example 7: The Headless Pastor

A pastor friend dreams that he is going to minister as a guest in a church. He arrives on time and sits up front, where the guest of honor would sit. The people are a bit unruly and disorganized, but everything seems okay. When it is time to announce the guest pastor, the senior pastor of the church comes to the pulpit without a head.

Focus, *Subfocus*, and *Important Details*

A pastor friend dreams that he is going to <u>minister as a guest</u> in a church. He arrives on time and sits up front, where the guest of honor would sit. The people are a bit <u>unruly</u> and <u>disorganized</u>, but everything seems okay. When it is time to announce the guest pastor, the senior pastor of the church comes to the pulpit without a head.

Symbols

Senior pastor = a senior pastor or leader

Headless = without authority or without Christ as the head

Minister as a guest = bringing a message to another group of people

Unruly and disorganized = literal

(The interpretation is on the next page.)

Interpretation

This is a prophetic warning dream about a situation in which you have a message to take to another congregation that you will find to be disorganized and lacking in authority, thus making it hard for you to be heard or recognized. The dream is offering insight about the upcoming situation so that you can prepare.

Interesting Follow-Up

When I later talked to the pastor and asked how the dream manifested, he said that soon after the dream during one of his guest speaking engagements, everything happened just like in the dream. He barely got a chance to speak because the people randomly interrupted the service. It was disorganized, and lacked unity and leadership. However, because of forewarning and lots of resulting prayer, he was prepared to handle it.

Note: This is an example of a mostly literal dream. Also, it is important that there is no judgment or accusation toward the church or pastor. The guest pastor was only given this information to prepare himself.

Example 8: Taking a Bubble Bath at Church

I am in an old-fashioned, white bathtub full of water with bubbles. The tub is sitting on a platform about three feet high in a room of my church. The walls and doors of the room are all glass. People are walking by and waving, saying hello, and even stopping for brief conversations. I do not feel embarrassed but am very glad for the bubbles that cover me.

Focus, *Subfocus*, and <u>*Important Details*</u>

I am in an old-fashioned, white bathtub full of <u>water</u> with <u>bubbles</u>. The tub is sitting on a <u>platform</u> about three feet high in a room of my church. The walls and doors of the room are all <u>glass</u>. People are walking by and waving, saying hello, and even stopping for brief conversations. I do not <u>feel</u> embarrassed but am very glad for the bubbles that cover me.

Symbols

Bathtub = a place of cleansing

Water = spirit; Holy Spirit, who cleanses us

Bubbles = open; vulnerable; joy

Platform = elevated; a place where you can be seen

Glass = clear; can see through

(The interpretation is on the next page.)

Interpretation

This is a direction dream showing that you will be given a platform to share and teach from your personal experiences in the church. You will be open and vulnerable to share the joy of cleansing where everyone will see and recognize what is happening. The Holy Spirit is using the church as a place to remove outer toxins of daily life and bring refreshing and cleansing to you in a safe and non-embarrassing environment.

Example 9: Thief in the Bedroom

I see a pastor friend sleeping in his bedroom at night. I watch a man dressed in black come in and steal the pastor's watch and wallet from the nightstand.

Focus, *Subfocus*, and *Important Details*

I see a pastor friend sleeping in his bedroom at night. I watch a man dressed in black come in and steal the pastor's watch and wallet from the nightstand.

Symbols

Pastor friend = literal friend or someone with same attributes

Man dressed in black (who steals) = enemy; thief

Sleeping = unaware

Watch = time

Wallet = money; finances; identity

(The interpretation is on the next page.)

Interpretation

This is a prophetic warning dream showing the plan of the enemy to steal someone's time, money, or identity. The person is likely unaware of the attack, and the Lord may be showing you this situation so that you can intercede for your friend.

Example 10: Working with Beth Moore

My sister Beth dreamed she is with Beth Moore in an office going through papers that contain teaching material. There are Bibles and notes piled in the room. It is like they are best friends working on something together (even though they have never met in real life).

Focus, Subfocus, and Important Details

My sister Beth dreamed she is with Beth Moore in an office going through papers that contain teaching material. There are Bibles and notes piled in the room. It is like they are best friends working on something together (even though they have never met in real life).

Symbols

Beth Moore = a strong and passionate leader in women's ministry

Teaching material and Bibles = the theme of the task at hand; teaching/learning/sharing God's Word

The name "Beth" = both women share the same name

Office = an appointment; role or responsibility

(The interpretation is on the next page.)

Interpretation

This is a calling dream to inform/confirm to the dreamer that she has a teaching gift to passionately share God's Word with many others.

Interesting Follow-Up

The dreamer, Beth Stewart, is the founder of *Triumphant Living* radio ministry and the CEO of Beth Stewart Ministries, which reaches over thirty nations. She speaks to many church groups, conferences, businesses, and organizations in the effort to bring hope and encouragement to help facilitate the fulfillment of destiny and God-given dreams within people.

LESSONS LEARNED

Over the many years that I have been interpreting dreams (or learning to do so), I have gleaned a few nuggets of insight and would like to share them with you for your journey.

Try to see the dream through the dreamer's eyes. John Paul Jackson taught that we should walk through the dream as if we are the dreamer to gain a visual perspective that will help us to interpret while connecting us to the dream and the dreamer.

Understand that some interpretations will be rejected. Not everybody will receive the interpretation you give them, either, because it does not bear witness in their spirit or because they want to deny the problem it addresses in their life. Some of the hardest interpretations to get across are those dealing with matters of the heart, especially in the area of dating and marriage. A woman who is desperate to find "the man of her dreams" is hard to convince that her dream of intimacy with a mysterious man is really the Lord desiring a deeper commitment or covenant relationship with her. They often forego the spiritual meaning of the dream for a literal one. In one extreme case, I had a lady, who was incredibly infatuated with a famous man, decide that her recurring dreams about him meant that it was fate for them to be together. Despite my multiple efforts to explain the symbolic meaning of the dreams to her, she packed up and traveled to act on the dream. I tried to explain to her the dream was symbolic rather than literal, but she was convinced in her mind and there was no stopping her. She literally went several states away in an attempt to connect with him. Needless to say, he was not what she was expecting and things did not turn out like she thought her dreams were indicating.

Disconnect yourself from the dreamer's dreams and responsibilities. An important lesson, learned over time, is disconnecting yourself from a perceived responsibility to the dreamer. I used to dread hearing negative dreams until I realized that I have nothing to do with it—in the same way that it is not the fault of the mailman that we receive bills. I had to come to the understanding that I did not give the dream, the dream and the message are not mine, I do not feel bad delivering the message, and I do not judge the dreamer for the message. Once we deliver the interpretation and pray for the dreamer, our job is done and we can move on, leaving the dream and its interpretation with the dreamer. Our responsibility is not to fix the dreamer or counsel them about the dream. The dreamer is accountable for it and has the duty of seeking the Father for more understanding or help.

Get feedback after providing interpretations. When you interpret your own, be sure to record the interpretation in your dream journal so that you can look back and note how it worked out. When working with other dreamers, it is important to get their feedback, too. It helps confirm whether you are on track. Ask them questions like whether the interpretation bears witness to them, or if you have the opportunity later, ask them how it played out in real life.

Seek feedback from trusted friends on your interpretations. Having a couple of friends skilled in discernment of dreams is helpful, especially in the beginning. As iron sharpens iron, so one person sharpens another.[78] Share dreams that need confirmation, especially if you are making an important life decision such as marriage, a geographical move, or a career change.

Practice is an ongoing and lifelong necessity. When it comes to giving dream interpretations to others, a lot of zeal with a little knowledge can be contagious but unfruitful or even harmful. To learn dream interpretation will require an investment of your time and resources. Look for Bible-based classes in dream interpretation or a church prophetic group (there are always dreamers in there). In addition, consider Christian websites where you can practice interpreting dreams. Dream interpretation is an area where you can always get better, but you never really "arrive." There is a scriptural reason for that. The Lord wants us to continually depend on Him, and if we think we already have all the answers, we tend to forget that. Be content with being a student rather than an expert, and always look for opportunities to practice.

Interpreting dreams for Christians is different than for nonbelievers. I learned this truth really fast when I started doing dream interpretation as part of street ministry. Most of the dreams have the same theme overall: salvation and deliverance. In general, dreams of unsaved people are usually warning dreams, and may include their dilapidated homes (their spiritual condition), thieves breaking in and stealing (the enemy comes to steal, kill, and destroy), or dark figures that are chasing them. They will commonly have dreams of their teeth falling out, meaning that they cannot seem to bite into the things of God and lack understanding/wisdom to chew on the Word. When ministering on the street, try to stay positive and be as encouraging as possible. Repeat the dream back to them, making sure you heard it correctly. (This also allows you time to think and ask the Holy Spirit to show you the meaning.) Because there is no time to write everything down and look up all the symbols, it is helpful to use a team approach and always have two to three people with you. Remember to keep the interpretation brief to help them remember it, and use language they will understand rather than Christian terms. (For example, instead of "revelation" you could say "you will see things clearly and gain fresh insight.") Use extra grace and love in the delivery of it.

RESOURCES

Because it can be hard to discern Bible-based dream interpretation resources versus New Age ones, I have created a list of resources that I personally use and endorse. This list is by no means exhaustive, but it provides a starting point for beginners.

Books

Understanding the Dreams You Dream, Revised and Expanded by Ira Milligan

The Seer: The Prophetic Power of Dreams, Visions, and Open Heavens by Jim Goll

Dreams and Visions: Understanding Your Dreams and How God Can Use Them to Speak to You Today by Jane Hamon

Understanding Your Dreams Now: Spiritual Dreams Interpretation by Doug Addison

Dream Encounters: Seeing Your Destiny from God's Perspective by Barbie Breathitt

Dreams: A Biblical Model of Interpretation by Zach Mapes and Jim Driscoll

Dream Interpretation Leaders and Their Websites

John Paul Jackson at www.streamsministries.com

Michael French at www.cahaba.org

Ira Milligan at www.servant-ministries.org

James Goll at www.encountersnetwork.com

UNIT 4:
DREAM DICTIONARY

The symbols in this dictionary are basic tools meant to start you thinking in terms of figurative and metaphoric dream language. They can be very helpful for building your dream vocabulary, but you need to be led by the Holy Spirit in order to apply them constructively to a specific dream.

ANIMALS

AARDVARK: Anteater; has nose in things; takes out the industrious, productive workers (i.e., ants); rids pests.

ADDER: See *Snake.*

ALLIGATOR/CROCODILE: Malicious speech; coldhearted, unapproachable person; keeps a low profile; verbally abusive (snaps at you if come near); agenda is to drag you down; uses its tail or slander for the "death roll" of tearing and twisting prey into pieces; big mouth, long powerful tail (symbolizing lies); hides below the surface; fear you'll be taken down in an area of life (finances, job, etc.); controls the environment through fear; attack is painful and requires time to recover; if attack is fatal, it could end your ministry or career. Baby alligators: issues are multiplying and grow quickly; showing signs of aggression and slander in the early stages; big issues are multiplying into small ones. "What a croc," meaning lies. A crocodile is similar to the alligator except it's more vicious.

ANCHOVIES: Offensive to some; something smells fishy; little fish with big impact (positive or negative); salty fish (increases thirst); schools of small fish are places of learning for youth. See Matt 5:13. See also *Fish.*

ANT: Small annoyances; drawn to spiritual food (picnics or places of service); wise, organized workers; industrious; teamwork, gather and store for the future; social network in colonies. See Pro 6:6.

ANTELOPE: Lovely, graceful gazelle; slender, shy, and timid; the image of feminine loveliness; swift-footedness. See 2 Sam 1:19, 2:18, 1 Chr 12:8, Song of Sol 4:5, 2:9, 2:17, 8:14.

APE: Acts like a beast; self-centered; going ape over something (i.e., excitement or anger); foolish ("big ape"); intimidating; powerful; among gifts to Solomon. See 1 Kings 10:22, 2 Chr 9:21. See also *Gorilla.*

ARMADILLO: Lives in protective armor; antisocial; harasser; destroyer; digs into things.

BADGER: Pestering person; badgering a witness in court is making accusations instead of asking questions; French name translates "digger."

BAT: Enjoys the dark places (i.e., caverns); rids insects; dark spirits controlling the atmosphere; batty/flighty personality; associated with witchcraft; night creature; vampire bats feed on blood; "blind as a bat." See Lev 11:19, Rev 6:16, Is 2:20.

BEAR: Angry or emotional confrontation from you or another if provoked; comes out of nowhere; financial hardship; hungry for what you have; aggressive; powerful; stalks you; if you stand up to it, it will lash out; declining market trend such as a bear market (claws pointing down/market goes down); confronting a fear; "bare necessities"; symbol for Russia or a government; "bear" a burden; possessive parent; intelligent; loves honey (the Word); resurrection (going into the darkness, coming out in the spring—new life); Mama protects her young; strength; symbol of a warrior; fishing skills. See Rev 13:2, 2 King 2:23, Dan 7:5. See also *Polar Bear*.

BEAVER: Busy as a beaver; industrious; diligent; skillful; engineering; blocks the flow; causes land damage for their own purpose. See Pro 10:4, 24:3.

BEES: Demonic harassment; create a "buzz"; stinging words; busy as a bee; gossip in the atmosphere; honeybees represent anointing; chase people off; cross-pollinate (i.e., carry ideas or things from place to place); queen can represent Jezebel spirit (i.e., everyone doing her bidding). See Deut 1:44, Ps 118:12, 1 Tim 5:13. See also *Honeybee*.

BIRD: Messenger; people; sacrifices; worshipers; angels; birds of a feather flock together; "free as a bird"; white birds–uplifting and inspiring; blackbirds–evil reports; dark thoughts over the mind; plans of the enemy circling you; carnal, sinful nature; negative person; songbirds–worship; freedom without restraint; rising above circumstances. See Is 46:11. See also *Buzzard, Chicken, Crane, Crow, Dove, Duck, Eagle, Flamingo, Goose, Hawk, Hen, Homing Pigeon, Hummingbird, Ostrich, Owl, Parrot, Peacock, Raven, Rooster, Seagull, Sparrow, Stork, Swan, Turkey,* and *Vulture*.

BLACK WIDOW: Feeling trapped; unforgiving situation; consumes mate (widow); gets what it needs, then kills; associated with witchcraft. See also *Spider.*

BOAR: Aggressive male swine; hunts for food; ravages the land; unclean; detestable in many customs; "boring." See Ps 80:13. See also *Pigs.*

BUFFALO: Intimidate; deceive, as in "buffalo" others into believing you; wild game; thick neck; great memory; unforgiving–will attack years after a person hurts them.

BULL: Stubborn/bullheaded; enemy; aggressive; positive market trends, such as bull market (horns that point up, the market goes up); dominating; stretching the truth; important for economy; bully; idol; sacrifice. See Heb 9:13, 10:4, Ps 22:12. See also *Cow* and *Ox.*

BUTTERFLY: Transformed life; metamorphosis from death to life; moved by the wind of the Holy Spirit; social butterfly; beautiful, fragile, and short-lived; not grounded (i.e., flutters from place to place). See 2 Cor 5:17, Rom 12:2. See also *Caterpillar.*

BUZZARD: Feeds off dead things; can be seen circling dying things; territorial; scavenger; "old buzzard" (contemptible). See Rev 18:2.

CAMEL: Burden bearer; getting over a hump; endures dry and hot conditions; a geographical location (esp. the East); economic resource; "the straw that broke the camel's back" (something building up until it breaks). See Gen 24:10 (for riding), 32:15 (for milk), Matt 3:4 (for hair into cloth).

CAT: Independent thinker; beloved pet; self-willed; one who is "catty" is insulting; a fickle friend (affectionate one minute and turns its back the next); curious about others' business ("curiosity killed the cat"); playful; moody; unable to speak or has no reply ("cat got your tongue"); exposed secret ("cat's out of the bag"); catfight (girl fight); "fight like cats and dogs"; black cat—associated with witchcraft. See also *Leopard, Lion, Panther,* and *Tiger.*

CATERPILLAR: Something or someone in the early stages of development (needs patience); going through a life change;

takes what it can; soulish issues; must die to self to live a transformed life (become a butterfly); hungry for more; desire for growth; potential for beauty. See Joel 2:25. See also *Butterfly*.

CHAMELEON: Changes personality based upon environment; conformity; blends in with the crowd; changes color (appearance) to display emotion. See Rom 12:2.

CHICKEN: Provision (i.e., meat and eggs); coward (being "chicken"); grounded (can't stay in the air or fly like other birds); "fowl/foul play"; "as a mother hen gathers and protects her brood under her wings so the Lord gathers His own." See Luke 13:34.

COW: Prosperity, provision, slow, laborious. Calf–immature; the choicest food (i.e., the fattened calf); prosperity; used for sacrifices; idol worship (Israelites made a calf of gold in the wilderness). See Ex 32:4, Deut 30:9, Luke 15:23, Ps 68:30. See also *Bull* and *Ox*.

CRAB: Cranky mood ("crabby"); hides in its shell when approached; claws that pinch; crab-walking (appears to move sideways).

CRANE: Shallow-water bird (doesn't get into deep spiritual things); straining your neck around to see; loner. See Jer 8:7.

CROCODILE: See *Alligator*.

CROW: Old, cranky person ("old crow"); associated with grief or sad times; thievery; "eat crow" (wrong about something that brings open humiliation); "as the crow flies" (in a straight line); crow about something (boast); wide binocular vision.

DEER: Graceful; gentle; timid; hinds feet are made for high places; pants for water as our soul thirsts for the Lord; someone or something dear to you; overcomes difficult places; surefooted. See Hab 3:19, 2 Sam 22:34, Pro 5:19, Ps 18:33, 42:1, 18:33.

DINOSAUR: Old belief system; extinct; ancient religious spirit; predator; big issue that should have died a long time ago; still doing something that seems extinct in our culture (e.g., long marriage; righteous life); outdated.

DOG: Friendship ("man's best friend"); watchman and protector ("watchdog"); those outside the kingdom; strife ("fight like cats and dogs"); wild or stray dog—refuses authority and lives on scraps; Hound dog—something following you around ("hounding you"); Sheepdog (protects the sheep); German shepherd (our Shepherd); Doberman (military/police); retriever (returns what was lost); bulldog (stubborn, bullheaded); pet dog—someone or something beloved. Dogs devoured Jezebel. See 1 Kings 21:23, Phil 3:2, Rev 22:15, Is 56:10, Job 30:1, 1 Sam 24:14, 2 Sam 3:8, 9:8, 16:9, Matt 15:26-27, 7:6.

DOLPHIN: Intelligent; trainable (i.e., to jump through hoops); always wears a smile; playful; amusing; will sometimes attack a porpoise/purpose for some unknown reason.

DONKEY: Stubborn; Jesus rode in on a donkey demonstrating humility; Balaam's donkey spoke when God opened its mouth; God uses foolish things to confound the wise; pack animal (carries burdens); slow; Eeyore's character—depressed. See 1 Cor 1:27, Num 22:28, Matt 21:5, Zech 9:9.

DOVE: Holy Spirit; peace; harmless; sacrifice used by the poor; messenger; love; gentle; rapid flight; faithful to one mate for life. See Matt 10:16, Ps 55:6, and 68:13.

DRAGON: Devil; false authority; demonic attack; end-time events symbol of China; fire-breather; dragon breath (foul talk). See Rev 20:2.

DRAGONFLY: Revelation from dark source (wordplay/flying dragon); positive in some cultures, so must consider context; old tales say if you see a dragonfly, beware of a snake.

DUCK: Loves the water ("like a duck takes to water"); "like a duck out of water" (out of your element); "duck" (keep a low profile); unity (fly in formation); target, as in "sitting duck"; allows insults to roll off its back; quack (medical fraud or inadequate); lame duck is someone who has lost their impact; "dead duck," as in trouble or doomed; "if it looks like a duck and walks like duck, then it's a duck" (you can call it by another name, but it is still a duck).

EAGLE: Prophetic (sees what others cannot see); eagle eyes (power of vision); Christ; United States; flies high in spirit; swift flight; eagle in golf (2 under par). See Deut 28:49, 2 Sam 1:23, Job 39:27, Ex 19:4.

ELEPHANT: Huge influence; big issue that everyone ignores ("elephant in the room"); prophet (big ears to hear and nose of discernment); memory issues ("an elephant never forgets"); stronghold in the spirit (an elephant sitting on you); stays with family; Republican party; elephant trunk can also be a trumpet or a voice; baby elephant is the beginning of something big; elephant charging you is a big issue coming at you.

FISH: Souls of men; evangelism; prospective believers; ichthus is the fish symbol (Jesus Christ is God's Son, Savior); something fishy (up to something). See Matt 4:19.

FLAMINGO: Thrives in social groups/colonies, their diet causes their color (i.e., it is evident what they are consuming); wader; tropical; Bahamas' national bird.

FLIES: Live off of dead things; false doctrine; Beelzebub ("lord of the flies"); carry disease; "dropping like flies" (sudden, rapid fall or death); "how time flies" (quickly passes). See Ecc 10:1.

FOX: Sly; sneaky; cunning; scheming; wants what you have; little foxes spoil the vine/your fruit; after the eggs; attractive lady. See Song of Sol 2:15, Neh 4:3, Lam 5:17, Ps 63:9, Luke 13:32.

FROG: Curses; plague; unclean spirits, lust; "frog in throat" (need to clear your throat); noisy complaints (croaking sounds). See Ex 8:2, Rev 16:13.

GOOSE: Member of a spiritual group; flying high; flock together; unity (fly in formation); prefer small bodies of water (smaller groups, conferences); on land they are noisy and destructive; "someone cooked your goose" (ruins your chances for success).

GIRAFFE: Pride; looks down on others; sticks their neck out for you; overseer; can get things normally out of reach.

GOAT: Unsaved; goat nation (not followers of Christ); walking in flesh rather than the spirit (perhaps doing good things with the wrong spirit); strong-willed; irritation ("get your goat"); self-willed; someone taking the blame for others and rejected (scapegoat); "you old goat." See Matt 25:32, Lev 16:10.

GORILLA: Control; can be calm and get along with other species; "guerilla" warfare; a group of gorillas is called a troop; each has individual fingerprints. See also *Ape*.

HAWK: Counterfeit of prophetic eagle; psychic; feeds off of others; Native American warrior symbol; "hawk-eyed" (watchful, sharp eyesight).

HEN: Mothering traits; protector like Christ or a mother/Church; allows others to feed off of them; "mad as a wet hen" (mature woman with angry temper). See Luke 13:34. See also *Chicken*.

HIPPO: Big mouth; territorial; will charge you; bossy; throws weight around, not caring who they hurt; dangerous around humans; allows others to feed off of them.

HOMING PIGEON: Messenger; angels bringing a message home; personal way of communication.

HONEYBEE: Sweet words; honey is anointing; stinging words get under your skin; a painful barbed stinger keeps stinging even when the bee is removed. See also *Bee*.

HORSE: Strength; power ("horsepower"); authority; a system of power; four apocalyptic horsemen (white, red [war], black [famine], pale [death]); "horsing around." See Rev 6:5, Am 8:11.

HUMMINGBIRD: Joyful (humming); fruitful–eats the nectar; tireless; busy; humming (from wings); tiny; quick; pleasant; blessings coming; fascinating. See also *Bird*.

HYENA: Mocking; making fun of; offensive; laughing sounds; strong but cowardly; lives in clans.

JELLYFISH: Stinging words; hidden below the surface; spineless; you can see through it; can still sting when dead, indicating long-lasting pain even when the offender is gone.

KANGAROO: Nurtures and protects what it carries; jumps in with both feet; boxes it out (males); "kangaroo court" (leans toward injustice and biased judgments); one who hides things in pockets. See 1 Cor 9:26.

KOALA: Something that looks cute and harmless but will attack when disturbed; Australia; sleeps about eighteen hours per day.

LAMB/SHEEP: Christians; Christ is the Lamb of God; sacrifice; innocence; Church; Israel; hear the shepherd's voice; sheep nations (followers of Christ); lie down in green pastures; "ewe" (wordplay for "you"); "black sheep of the family"; economic resource (wool, meat, milk). See Jn 10:27, Gen 4:3–4, Matt 25:33, Ps 23:2. See also *Ram.*

LEOPARD: Leader–preys on the weak and vulnerable; likes to be among trees (i.e., leadership); smallest of the big cats but most effective; dangerous predator; endangered (protected); loner; works fast; goes for the jugular vein (quick kill); hidden danger; if caged, the danger is contained and held back from you; "can't change its spots" (will never change). See Jer 5:6.

LICE: Negative or unclean thoughts; curse (third plague of Egypt); parasites (covers your hair/thinking); hard to get rid of; multiplies, and negativity can transfer to others. See Ex 16:20, Ps 105:31.

LION: King Jesus; tribe of Judah/Jesus; authority; roars over territory; lioness is the bride of Christ/Church; king; valiant; strength; boldness; ferocity; devourer; your adversary–"the devil as a roaring lion." See Rev 5:4–5, 1 Pet 5:8, Jud 14:18, 2 Sam 17:10, Ps 7:2, 10:9, 17:12, 104:21, Lam 3:10, Job 4:10, Is 31:4, Gen 49:9, Deut 33:22, 1 Chr 12:8, Pro 19:12, Hos 5:14, 1 Pet 5:8, 1 King 7:29&36, 10:19.

LOBSTER: In the deep things; bottom dweller; equipped to hold on; delicacy; hard shell; lives long life (up to 100 years); unclean. See Lev 11:10.

LOCUST: Judgment; curse; power to destroy; spiritual attack on possessions or health; John the Baptist ate locusts and honey. See Ex 10:14, Rev 9:3, 9:7–10, Joel 1:4, Mark 1:6.

MAGGOT: Lives off dead things; rotting; larvae becomes a fly; reproach; curse. See Ex 16:20, Ps 22:6, Acts 12:23.

MICE/MOUSE: Small issues; pests; timid; unclean devourer; curse. See 1 Sam 6:5, Lev 11:29. See also *Rat.*

MONKEY: Playing around ("monkey" around/"monkey business"); "monkey on your back" (burden, addiction, hard to get rid of).

MOOSE: Large and clumsy in man-made environments; have a lot hanging on your head; if animated, then Bullwinkle characteristics.

MOSQUITOES: Small irritations get under your skin; stinging words that leave discomfort afterward; bloodsucker; disease carrier; lay eggs in water; buzzing in your ear (gossip).

MOTH: Destroys coverings (or mantles); hidden deterioration of earthly treasures. See Matt 6:19.

OCTOPUS: Control; manipulation; Jezebel spirit (i.e., Ursula); multitasker; someone who has their hands in everything; many arms.

OSTRICH: Fast runner; strength in the legs; a bird that cannot fly; heartless and cruel; fights with feet. See Job 39:13–17, Lam 4:3. See also *Bird*.

OWL: Earthly wisdom; analytical; an idea; someone inquisitive–asking who; bird of the night; getting revelation from the dark side; curse. See Is 34:13.

OX: Strong worker ("strong as an ox"); pioneering; ploughs the field for harvest; groundbreaker; beast of burden. See 1 Sam 14:14, Hos 10:11.

PANTHER/JAGUAR: Black; stealth; operates in high-level witchcraft.

PARROT: Gossip; imitator; repeats what it hears. See Ecc 10:20.

PEACOCK: Pride ("proud as a peacock"); beautiful but vain; arrogant; feathers appear to have eyes; colorful; vibrant. See Rev 4:8.

PENGUIN: Discernment (it's black or white); protector of youth; keeping your cool; letter of the law.

PIG: Unclean; backslider (i.e., prodigal son); unbeliever; glutton ("pig out"); "when pigs fly" (never); provision (ham); evil spirits; demons; hypocrite; destroyer; idolater. See 2 Pet 2:22, Luke 8:33.

PIRANHAS: Deadly as a group; feeding frenzy; eat away at things in their path; small things with big bites; work together.

POLAR BEAR: Religious spirit (white appearance is deceiving); appears righteous but is spiritually cold; false prophet; coldhearted; huge issue creating fear; endangered; global warming awareness; two polar bears could mean bipolar actions; someone or something that polarizes the atmosphere. See also *Bear.*

PUPPY: New friendship or commitment that requires time and care; will mature and grow in time to be a loyal friend; young or immature person (needs training). See Pro 17:17. See also *Dog.*

RABBIT: Multiplication (ideas, business growth); lust; fast growth; "pull a rabbit out of a hat"; pagan rituals/fertility; white rabbit running late; timid. See Pro 20:21.

RACCOON: Bandit; thief; masking or hiding something; takes whatever it can get for itself; leaves a big mess behind; pursuit of shiny things. See Pro 4:16.

RAM: Offering; Christ (as sacrifice and leader); force; ramming something; using head to get one's way; replacement sacrifice. See 1 Sam 15:2, Dan 8:20.

RAT: Untrustworthy; poor moral character; something detestable in your surroundings; transmits disease; a person "is a rat" if they are underhanded and deceptive; mischief (the name for a group of rats); "rat you out"; intelligent; pet issue; object of experiments; packrat (stores things it does not need). See Is 66:17. See also *Mouse.*

RAVEN: Dark messages; evil intentions; worldly provision (ravens fed Elijah); highly intelligent; mysterious. See 1 King 17:4. See also *Bird.*

RHINO: Harsh; throws weight around; angry; powerful; its charge tries to gouge you and can be bloody; hateful.

ROACH: Uncleanliness in one's life; hidden sins multiplying; infestation; difficult to detect; spreads germs and allergens; drugs (marijuana); hides from the light.

ROOSTER: Sounds the alarm; new beginning; a new day is coming; denial; crowing (bragging). See Mark 14:30.

SCORPION: Stinging tails/tales causing great pain; unfaithful friend; black or white magic; we are given power over them. See Luke 10:19, 1 Cor 15:56, Rom 7:23.

SEAGULL: Messenger; moves on the wind of the Spirit; predator; can represent a religious person who is self-seeking and leaves messes behind. See also *Bird*.

SEALS: Deep things of God; highly intelligent; teachable/entertaining; slippery; Navy Seals (mentally and physically sharp); below-the-surface operation; wordplay on "seals" (as in signets); seven seals described in Revelation; end-time prophecy. See Rev 6.

SHARK: Predator that tries to take you under with its mouth (vicious words); unseen threat; exploits the finances of the weak ("loan shark"); scammer; swindler; double-dealer; con artist.

SKUNK: Creates a "stink" that everyone notices; controversial views (black and white), but not well accepted (i.e., doctor-assisted suicide, abortion, cloning); offensive; people want to avoid a confrontation with it; social outcast; something you may do that drives people away; beat badly in competition.

SLOTH: Lazy; slow; sluggard; one of seven deadly sins. See Pro 18:9, Ecc 10:18, Pro 18:9, 1 Tim 5:8.

SNAIL: Untimely; slow-moving; has protection of a shell/covering; as one who doesn't see the sun and fades away. See Ps 58:8.

SNAKES: Lies; satan (father of lies) in the Garden of Eden; curse; deception; scheming; demon; danger; releasing poisonous words/venom; if bitten can cause prolonged pain; long tales about you; healing (caduceus). White snake—religious spirit or white lies. Black snake—lies sent from the enemy; python—someone suffocating the life out of you; rattlesnake—creates fear with sound; copperhead—dealing with money. See Gen 3:14, 49:17, Am 5:19, Pro 23:32, Ps 58:4, 91:13, 140:3, Num 21:9, Matt 12:34, Jer 8:17.

SPARROW: God watches over the small and ordinary things. See Matt 10:29–31, Luke 12:7.

SPIDER: Something trying to entrap you that can eventually kill you (addictions, hatred); spins a web; demonic; occult; something seemingly small and difficult to see, but venomous; stinging words; creates fear; feeling of being walked all over (eight legs). See Is 59:4–5.

SQUIRREL: Stock up for times ahead ("squirrel away"); practical; nutty or hyper character ("squirrelly").

STORK: Appointed time; expecting something new; very caring to young ones and parents; new experience. See Jer 8:7.

SWAN: Elegant; "graceful as a swan"; freedom from distractions; comes from ugly duckling (famous fairy tale); "swan song" (last saying before dying).

TIGER: Someone you know who is a dangerous stalker; stripes influence the soul or mind; aggressive; "grab a tiger by the tail" (grab something dangerous and impossible to manage).

TURKEY: Stubborn and stiff-necked; "talk turkey" (talk plainly/frankly); stop "cold turkey"; Thanksgiving.

TURTLE: Withdrawn; insecure; peace; will not confront issues; slow but eventually will get there (tortoise and the hare–"slow and steady wins the race"); safe; old religious system.

VULTURE: Death; greed; feeds on dead things and the vulnerable (inheritance after a death). See Matt 24:28. See also *Buzzard*.

WEASEL: Clever teller of secrets; betrayal; self-gain; shifty and scheming person who will do whatever it takes to get out of something ("weasel out of").

WHALE: Huge influence or impact; can be a prominent person or a potentially large problem ("makes waves"); dangerous predator.

WOLF: Predator (after the sheep); devourer; false prophet; deceptive minister or governor ("wolf in sheep's clothing"–evil minister); person seeking their own gain; womanizer; loner ("lone wolf"); unwanted. See Matt 7:15, Acts 20:29–30.

WORM: Devourer; burrows inside; not easily seen; bait for lost souls; hidden damage; something has "wormed its way into your life." See Acts 12:23, Jon 4:7.

ZEBRA: Discernment; black-and-white thinking; leader who struggles with multiple issues; afflicted.

COLORS & METALS

AMBER: God's glory; fire; God's presence in holiness or judgment; throne of God; wisdom; holy purification; Temple of God; idolatry; contamination. See Ez 1:4, 1:27–28, 8:22, 2 Cor 4:6, Heb 12:29, Ex 3:2, Rev 21:23, Gen 19:24, 2 King 1:10–14, Is 66:15, 2 Thes 1:7–8.

AQUA: Mixture of blue and green; growth; prosperity; prophetic; evangelism outreach.

BABY BLUE: Developing or learning revelation; sapphire; influence; male child. See Ex 23:3–8, 24:10, Ez 1:26, 10:1, Num 15:38.

BLACK: Hidden; sin; lack; witchcraft; disease; enemy; famine (the third seal of famine and the black horse); blindness; formal event (i.e., black tie, weddings, funeral, preaching, speeches); death; grief/sorrow; darkness. See Gen 1:4, Jn 1:5, 2 Pet 2:17, Lev 13:37, Song of Sol 1:5–6, 5:11, Ps 18:9&11, Rev 6:5, Pro 7:6–9, Lam 5:10, Job 30:30, 6:15–16, 3:5, Jer 14:2, Eph 4:18.

BLUE: Revelation from God; communion and intimacy with Christ; heavenly; "the blues" (depression); prophet (revelation); authority; dominant color of the robe of Israel's high priest; blue cord to remember His commands; Holy Spirit; the Word; holy articles in the tabernacle were covered in blue when moved. See 2 Chr 3:14, Num 4:5–7, 15:38–40, Ex 26:1, Jn 14:26.

BRASS: Strength; judgment; hypocrisy; self-justification; tarnish; Word of God; word of man; man's tradition; fake; hardness; stronghold; brassy; noisy; brass section. See Num 21:9, Rev 1:15, 1 Cor 13:1, 2 Cor 12:10, Eph 6:16, Is 48:4.

BRONZE: Strength; fire of testing; judgment on sin. See Mic 4:13.

BROWN: Humility; missions; compassion; earthly; humanistic; pastoral; messenger; work; man's works; dead works; death (opposite of green). See 1 Pet 1:24, Ps 37:2.

BURGUNDY: Community; communion; stranded or deserted ("marooned").

COPPER: Monetary value; high value for utility; finances; police. See Deut 8:9, Mark 3:12.

CRIMSON: Sacrifice for sin; Jesus' shed blood; cleansing of sins; Passover. See Gen 9:4–5, Deut 12:23, 1 King 2:5, Heb 9:22, 1 Jn 1:7, Matt 26:28, Rom 5:9, Rev 1:5.

GOLD: Glory; prosperity; refined by trials and fire; holiness; seal; wisdom; truth; something precious; righteous; self-glorification; used for idol worship and the unholy; refined; truth; precious; righteous; seal; honor; great value; idolatry. See Rev 3:18, 1 Cor 3:12.

GRAY: Mixture of black and white; wisdom; mature; uncertainty or undefined ("gray area"); mind ("gray matter") not the spirit; confused; unseen; weakness; mourning/ashes; misperception; unknown; obscure; death; dreariness ("gray skies"). See Pro 16:31, Hos 7:9.

GREEN: Life; growth; conscience; prosperity; renewal; "go" (i.e., green light); evergreen/eternal life; fruitful and thriving; fresh; undefiled; harvest; frailty; rest; jealousy ("green with envy"); short-lived/fading. See Matt 3:10, Song of Sol 1:16, Luke 23:31, Ps 23:2, 37:2, 123, Hos 14:8, Ez 17:24, Job 15:31-32, Pro 11:28, Jer 11:16, 17:8, Luke 23:31, 1 Pet 2:4,, Is 15:6.

IRON: Strength; "iron sharpens iron" (we sharpen each other); bondage (placed in irons); iron furnace/trial; heavens as iron/closed; power; invincible; stronghold; strong-willed; stubborn; yoke of iron; labor tools; rule with a rod of iron (correction). See Dan 2:40–41, Is 48:4, Deut 28:48, Lev 26:19, 2 Sam 12:31, Jer 28:14, Pro 27:17, Rev 2:27.

LEAD: Heavy; judgment; sin; weight; burden; poisonous; wordplay "led." See Ex 15:10, Zech 5:8.

MAGENTA: Emotions; giving; love or hate.

NEON: Message trying to get your attention; reflects black light (dark revelation); symbolic of nightlife; soulish dreams; unsanctified place.

ORANGE: Perseverance; stubborn; danger/caution ahead (used on roadways); negative or positive power; courage; strong-willed; evil (associated with Halloween); first stone in third row of breastplate of Aaron (jacinth); companionship. See Pro 6:27, Luke 12:49&53, Matt 5:22.

PASTELS: Something developing that is immature now; soft, subtle, and innocent; fading; pale (white added).

PINK: Mixture of red and white; childlike innocence; faith; love; a heart after God; feminine/girl; passionate heart; heart of flesh; immature. See 2 Cor 11:2, Ez 36:26.

PLUM: Mixture of red and purple; richness; abundance; infilling of Holy Spirit.

PURPLE: Mixture of red and blue; royalty; authority; wealth; kingship; false authority. See Lam 4:5, Jud 8:26, Jn 19:2&5, Acts 16:14, Rev 17:4, Is 6:5–7, Luke 20:46.

RAINBOW: Covenant; promise; gay pride flag. See Gen 9:13.

RED: Wisdom; anointing; power; blood/life atonement; sacrifice; remission of sin; covenant; power; passion (good or bad); anger; war; bloodshed (with the second seal there went out a red horse); death; destruction; "red light district"; prostitution. See Nah 2:3, Is 11:2, 63:2–3, 2 King 3:22, Rev 6:3–4, 12:3, Matt 27:28, Is 1:18.

SILVER: Redemption/restoration; salvation; wisdom (hair); mercy; grace; privileged ("silver spoon/cup"); riches; valor; affliction; slavery; Judas betrayed Jesus for thirty pieces of silver; words of the Lord are like purified silver; silver and gold vessels are in house of God; a word fitly spoken is like settings of silver; two trumpets to summon congregation; corruptible; idols. See Jn 17:3, Ps 12:6, Pro 2:3–4, Matt 26:15, Ezra 6:5, Pro 25:11, Num 10:2, 1 Pet 1:18, Rev 9:20. See also *Gray*.

STEEL: Strength; "man of steel"; "nerves of steel." See also *Iron*.

TIN: Impurity; lower status. See Is 1:25, Ez 22:18.

TURQUOISE: Mixture of blue, green, and white; combination of revelation, discerning, understanding; righteousness/ holiness. See also *Aqua*.

VIOLET: Mixture of purple and white; early stages of authority and leadership; beauty; peace; creativity; royalty. See also *Purple.*

WHITE: Holy; purity (without spot or mixture); glory; light; the great white throne; righteousness; angels; untarnished; consecrated; sanctified; divine; false religion; religious spirit; false purity; white on something evil is a cover-up. See Is 1:18, Dan 7:9, Jn 4:35, Mark 16:4, Rev 6:2, 7:9, 19:8–11, 19:14, 3:4–5, 15:6.

YELLOW: Renewed mind/intellectual pride; glory of God; honor; courage; hope (yellow ribbon); coward ("yellow belly"); gift/Son (sun) of God; caution light; sickness/disease. See Ps 68:13, Pro 19:14, Eph 2:7, Ex 35:6.

NUMBERS

1: God; first; unity; new beginning; single; first commandment is greatest; one body and one spirit; one faith; one baptism; One who is above all; looking out for number one (you). See Matt 22:37–38, Deut 6:4, Jn 10:30, Eph 4:4–6.

2: Divide/separate (God divided the waters from the heavens on second day of creation, parable of two in a field and one will be taken); judgment of God–second death in the lake of fire (separation from God); double (thief must pay back double, double anointing of Elisha); witness (disciples sent two by two, two witnesses establish truth); partnership; multiplication; two cherubim guarded the Ark of the Covenant. See Gen 1:7, Ex 22:7, 25:22, 2 King 2:9, Matt 22:37–40, 24:40, 25:32, 26:60, Mark 6:7, Luke 10:12, 2 Cor 13:1, Rev 11:3, 21:8.

3: Divine Trinity; completion (Jesus' ministry completed in three years); resurrection (Jesus was buried and raised the third day, as Jonah was three days and nights in the belly of the fish, Jesus was three days in the grave); divine perfection; darkness covered the earth for three hours before Jesus died on the cross; angels sing "Holy, Holy, Holy" around the throne; three aspects of time (i.e., past, present, future). See Luke 13:7, Matt 12:40, 28:19, 1 Cor 15:4, Is 6:3, Mark 15:33.

4: Creative works; rulership; earthly; on the fourth day of creation, God made two lights to rule the day and night; four gospels (Matthew, Mark, Luke, John); four directions (N, S, E, W); four seasons; four angels at the four corners of earth holding back the four winds; four rivers flowing from Eden; four types of soil/hearts (wayside, stony, thorny, good ground); four living creatures with four faces and four wings; sheet with four corners symbolizes the gospel going to all the Gentiles; after Jesus' death His clothes were divided by four men into four parts; four horsemen of the apocalypse released when Jesus opened the first four seals (horses were white, red, black, pale), the fourth horseman having power to kill a fourth of the earth; Daniel saw four great beasts that were four kings that will rise from the earth. See Gen 1:16, 2:10–14, Rev 6:1–8, 7:1, Matt 13:3–9, Acts 10:11, Jn 19:23, Dan 7:17.

5: God's grace; law; favor; blessing; calling; fivefold ministry (apostle, prophet, evangelist, pastor, teacher); Book of the Law is the first five books of the Old Testament; first five books of the New Testament are about grace; five wise virgins and five foolish ones; five barley loaves used to feed the 5,000; five books of the five Levitical offerings; Benjamin's portion was five times that of his brothers; David chose five stones for Goliath; the tabernacle had five curtains, five bars, five pillars; the altar was five cubits long and wide. See Ex 26, Gen 1:20, 43:34, Rom 6:14, Lev 1–5.

6: Works of the flesh; carnal nature; idolatry; work six days and rest the seventh; man and woman were created on the sixth day; man's weakness as opposed to strength through Christ; Hebrew slaves worked six years; the land was worked and harvested six years; Jesus turned six pots of water into wine; six cities of refuge given to the Levites for the manslayer to flee; six wings of seraphs and cherubim (three pairs); sixth seal is judgment. See Ex 35:2, Num 35:6, Dan 3:1, Rev 6:12.

7: God's fulfillment; completion; accomplished works; rest; seventh day is God's Sabbath rest from completed work of creation; seven days in a week; God's Word is pure, like silver purified seven times in the fire; seven annual Holy Days; seven stars in Jesus' right hand; seven angels of the seven churches, seven golden lampstands; seven spirits of God; seven seals opened by Jesus; seven angels; seven trumpets; seven crowns; seven plagues, seven thunders; Jesus tells Peter to forgive seven times seventy; Hebrew slaves were to be set free in the seventh year; Israelites marched around Jericho for seven days and seven times on the seventh day; the land is to rest every seven years; seven loaves of bread were multiplied; seven days in the Feast of Unleavened Bread observing the Israelites coming out of bondage in Egypt; seven letters written to the seven churches by John while exiled on Patmos; seven spirits before His throne; seven golden bowls; seven hills; seven kings; the lamb seen by John had seven horns, seven eyes, and seven spirits; seven heads; seven thousand people. See Rev 1:12, 1:16, 1:20, 2:1, 3:1, 3:22, 4:5, 5:6, 6:1–17, 8:2–6, 10:3–4, 11:13, 12:3, 13:1, 15:1–8, 17:3, 17:7, 17:9–11, 21:9, Gen 2:3, Ps 12:6, Matt 18:22, Ex 21:2, 34:18.

8: New beginning; circumcised heart (remove foreskin of heart, sealed with righteousness); teacher; new order of creation after seventh day; eight people saved from the flood; New Testament written by eight men; something completed; has come to fullness; circumcision of males occurred on the eighth day representing a new generation. See Gen 17:12, Num 29:35, 2 King 22:1, Jer 4:4.

9: Full maturity/fruitfulness (nine fruits of the Spirit; nine months of pregnancy); new season; end of a cycle; gifts of the Spirit; prayer; last hour of pain and suffering; judgment; divine completion; evangelism; conclusion; fullness of time; harvest; finality of one event to open the way for the new; nine generations from Adam to Noah; nine is the last single digit; Cornelius received salvation as first recorded Gentile on the ninth hour. See Matt 27:46, Gal 5:22–23, 1 Cor 12:8–10, Acts 3:11, 10:30.

10: Law; order; government; pastor; Ten Commandments; tithe is one-tenth; ten worldly government systems represented by the toes of the statue; testing; wise and foolish virgins; ten plagues sent to Egypt; ten tribes make up the northern kingdom; Boaz took ten elders of the city as judges; a leader was put over ten people and another leader over ten leaders; starting something new and doing things differently; ten curtains made up the tabernacle. See Ex 20:1–17, 18:21, 18:25, 34:28, 36:8, Dan 2, 1 Kings 11:31–35, Ruth 4:2, Deut 1:15.

11: Transition, prophetic anointing, revelation; judgment; confusion; disorder; eleven is an imperfect number before the twelfth divine order; chaos, antichrist is the eleventh horn; eleventh hour; incomplete; Matthias replaced Judas when there were eleven disciples; Joseph worked eleven years in Potiphar's household; King Zedekiah ruled wickedly for eleven years. See Jer 52:1–11, Dan 7:7–8, 1 Cor 13:9–10, Rev 7.

12: Divine government; apostle; order; completion; twelve apostles; twelve tribes of Israel; twelve judges; twelve months in a year; twelve on a court jury; New Jerusalem has twelve gates with twelve angels at the gates with names of the twelve tribes inscribed on them; twelve foundations of the wall of the city with the names of the twelve apostles on them; twelve fruits on the Tree of Life; twelve stones in the breastplate representing the twelve tribes of Israel; Joshua called twelve men from the twelve tribes to shoulder twelve stones from the middle of the Jordan; Abraham's sons, Ishmael and Jacob, both had twelve sons; the Church Bride wears a crown with twelve stars. See Rev 12, 22:2, Ex 39:14, Josh 4:4.

13: Rebellion; corruption; the wealth of the wicked is laid up for the righteous; Jericho was destroyed after Israelites circled it thirteen times; Nimrod was the thirteenth generation of Noah's son Ham; a baker's dozen; blessing in hard times. See Gen 14:4, Josh 6, Pro 13:22.

14: Double anointing (two sevens); deliverance; Passover; fourteen generations from Abraham to David; fourteen generations from David until the captivity in Babylon; fourteen generations from captivity until Christ; Jacob worked for Laban fourteen years for his wives (seven years for Leah and seven years for Rachel). See Matt 1:1–17.

15: Mercy; spiritual order; salvation; fifteen judges in Israel; God gave Hezekiah fifteen more years; freedom; set captives free. See Is 38:4–5.

16: Renewed relations; love; sixteen characteristics of love; sweet sixteen. See 1 Cor 13:4–8.

17: Triumph over trial; order; new life; Noah's ark rested on the seventeenth day of the seventh month.

18: Freedom/coming out of oppression; Israelites were in bondage and oppressed eighteen years in the Promised Land; a woman bent over with a spirit of infirmity for eighteen years was healed by Jesus; hope; ending a season of hardship. See Luke 13:11–13, Jud 3:12; 10:8.

20: Redemption; Jacob received redemption after twenty years of labor for Laban; Israelites who were destined to forty years in the wilderness at the age of twenty years or below were later allowed to enter the Promised Land; age for military service; twenty is a "score." See Num 1:3, Lev 27:3.

21: Resistance; prince of the Persian kingdom resisted Daniel twenty-one days; resistance to God's laws; twenty-one epistles in the New Testament. See Dan 10:13, 2 Tim 3:1–5.

24: Priesthood; worship; surrounding the throne are twenty-four other thrones, and seated on them are twenty-four elders. See Rev 4:4.

25: Begin ministry; repentance and forgiveness of sins; Levites began to serve at the age of twenty-five.

27: Evangelism; twenty-seven books in the New Testament.

30: Calling; prepared to enter ministry (Jesus and Aaronic priests, David began his reign over Israel); betrayal; Judas betrayed Jesus for thirty pieces of silver. See Num 4:3, 2 Sam 5:4, Luke 3:23.

33: Promise; Christ died at age of thirty-three; King David ruled over united Israel nation thirty-three years. See 1 King 2:11.

37: Bible; the Word of God.

38: Slavery; bondage. See Deut 2:14, Jn 5:5.

39: Healing (by Jesus' thirty-nine stripes). See Is 53:5.

40: Trials; testing; a generation; probation period; Noah in the flood forty days; Moses spent forty years in the wilderness with the Israelites to humble them and prove what was in their hearts; Moses was forty years old when he left Egypt and waited forty more years for his ministry; Moses died at 120 (40 x 3), the Ten Commandments were received by Moses after forty days on Mount Sinai (after breaking the tablets he returned another forty days); Saul, David, and Solomon reigned forty years as the first kings of Israel; Eli judged Israel forty years; for forty days Jesus fasted and was tested in the wilderness; it rained for forty days during the flood. See Gen 7:4, Deut 1:3, 8:2, 1 Sam 4:18, 2 Sam 5:5, 2 Chr 9:30, Acts 7:30.

42: Rebellion, tribulation; reign of the antichrist (forty-two months). See Dan 7:25, Rev 11:2, 12:5, 13:5.

50: Jubilee; Pentecost; liberty; reunited; set free from debt; celebration; feasts; Pentecost occurred fifty days after Christ's resurrection. See Ex 19:1, Lev 25:10, Acts 2.

52: Weeks in a year.

60: Pride; flesh; complete; Nebuchadnezzar's statue was sixty cubits high. See Dan 3:1.

66: Idolatry.

70: Order; judges/rulers; seventy elders were appointed by Moses; mourning (seventy days of mourning for Jacob); seventy souls went into Egypt; lifespan; seventy weeks of Daniel; exile; punishment; captivity; Israel spent seventy years captive in Babylon. See Jer 29:10, Dan 9:2, Ex 1:5, 15:27, Ps 90:10, Num 11:25, Luke 10:1.

80: Strong, full life; if strength endures. See Ps 90:10.

99: Incomplete; one sheep lost made the flock of ninety-nine incomplete until it was found; prodigal son. See Matt 18:12.

100: Completeness; promise; a complete flock was 100 sheep with none missing; children of promise; Abraham was 100 years old when Isaac was born to him; hundredfold blessing; Obadiah hid 100 prophets from Jezebel. See Gen 21:5, Luke 8:8, Matt 13:8, Mark 4:20.

120: God gave man 120 years for full life; waiting; timing of the Lord; Moses died at 120 years of age. See Gen 6:3.

144: Life guided by the Spirit; the wall of the city of God was 144 cubits thick. See Rev 21:17.

153: Fish in the net; evangelism. See Jn 21:11.

180: Repent; turn and go the other way (180-degree turn). See Pro 4:15.

200: Insufficiency; inadequate. See 2 Sam 14:26, Josh 7:21, Jn 6:7.

300: God's chosen remnant; valiant men in Gideon's army; deliverance; God's strength shown in our weakness. See Jud 7, 8, 15:4, Gen 5:22, 6:15, Jud 7:7.

360: To come full circle.

365: Enoch was 365 years old when God took him; 365 days in a year. See Gen 5:24.

390: Burden of Israel's sins. See Ez 4:5.

400: Fulfillment of time; 400 years of Israelites in Egypt; 400 years of silence between Old Testament and New Testament; Sarah's burial place cost 400 shekels. See Gen 23:3, Acts 7:6.

600: War. See Jud 18:11, 16–17.

666: Spirit of antichrist; mark of the beast; end times. See Rev 13:18.

700: Choice warriors; accuracy in battle. See Jud 20:15–16.

777: Christ.

911: Urgent situation; requiring assistance; a call for help to someone equipped and trained.

930: Age of Adam; number of years Adam lived. See Gen 3:5.

969: Number of years Methuselah lived. See Gen 5:27.

1,000: Complete glory of the Father; millennial reign; one day to God is 1,000 years to man. See Rev 20:5.

2,000: Church Age ending; resurrection; distance between man and the ark. See Josh 3:4.

7,000: Remnant (the righteous). See 1 King 19:18.

10,000: Innumerable (thousands and thousands and ten thousand times ten thousand stood before the throne and the books were open). See Dan 7:10, Rev 5:11.

12,000: The Lord's army. See Rev 7:5–8.

144,000: Remnant; numbered in Israel; number of martyrs. See Rev 14:3.

PEOPLE & OCCUPATIONS

ACTOR: Entertainer; acting out or making a dramatic production of a matter; pretending to be someone else but not the true nature; could represent someone with similar characteristics, qualities, or appearance.

APPRENTICE: Training; starting at the bottom to learn a trade.

ARAB: Associated with Middle East or Arab nation.

ARCHAEOLOGIST: Digging into history or the past.

ARCHITECT: God working out our plans; planning for future development; designer; overseer. See Job 38:4–6, Jer 29:11.

ASSISTANT: Holy Spirit; angel; helper. See Ps 121:2, Is 41:13.

ATTORNEY: Jesus; advocate; debate; counselor; pleading your case; presents the facts. See Luke 10:25.

BABY: Something new coming; new idea; early stages of ministry; career; project requiring nurturing and care; gift from God; literal baby; spiritually immature, innocent, new idea or skill that takes time to develop; twins–double blessing; extra work but worth it; baby boy–leadership ministry, apostolic, masculine qualities such as dominance; baby girl–birthing a new ministry involving prophetic and power gifts; feminine qualities of sensitivity toward others; subordination. See Is 42:9, Ps 127:3, 1 Cor 3:1, 1 Pet 2:2, Jam 1:14–15.

BAKER: Minister; prepares spiritual food for others; makes things sweet; creative/skilled; works leaven into the dough (works). See Pro 23:1–3.

BANDIT: Warning that the enemy is going to try to steal from your resources. See Jn 10:10, Hos 7:1.

BANK TELLER: Giving finances; favor; giving a prophetic word ("teller").

BANKER: Christ; financial advisor; handles investments and security for the future; ability to give favor and open doors of opportunity.

BEST FRIEND: Jesus (sticks closer than a brother); has your back; loves at all times; literal; the closest person to you. See Jn 15:15, Pro 18:24, 17:17.

BODYBUILDER: Building up the Body of Christ; gaining spiritual strength; strongman (could be a stronghold); building physical muscles; protection. See 1 Tim 4:8, Luke 11:21.

BOSS: Christ; authority figures in one's life; spiritual leader. See Rom 13:1, Pro 29:2, Col 3:22–25.

BRIDE: The Church; New Jerusalem; set apart for Christ in a covenant relationship; yoked with believers; wife-to-be. See Eph 5:31–32, 2 Cor 6:14, Is 62:5, Rev 21:2, 21:9.

BRIDEGROOM: Christ; husband-to-be. See Matt 9:15, 1 Tim 2:5.

BROTHER: Christian brother; spiritual tie; similar to you or your brother; male figure close and trusted; Jesus, a friend who sticks closer than a brother; mentor; literal. See Pro 18:24, Matt 25:40, Rom 2:1, 14:10, Heb 13:3.

BROTHER-IN-LAW: Literal; someone "in the law"; legalism; someone grafted into the family; not a blood relative. See Col 2:20–23.

BURGLAR: Enemy invading personal life; spiritual sabotage; takes what is precious to you; enemy comes to steal, kill, and destroy. See Jn 10:10, Pro 23:28.

CAPTAIN: Christ; leader; commander; head of. See Num 31:48, Heb 2:10.

CARPENTER: Jesus; person who builds character in others; literal builder; a work-in-progress; laborer. See Mark 6:3.

CELEBRITY: An aspect of your personality; qualities, opinions, or style; idolatry; high profile; person of influence in a region or community. See also *Actor.*

CEO: God.

CHEERLEADER: Motivator; supporter on your side; wants you to win.

CHEF: Minister; master at making spiritual food palatable and serving others.

CHILDREN: Next generation; blessed gift requiring teaching and loving care; young in the Lord; growing ministry (e.g., age of child can symbolize age of ministry); heritage of the Lord; arrows. See Ps 127:3, 127:4.

CHINESE: Ministry to reach China; eastern religion influence.

CHIROPRACTOR: Christ as healer; brings alignment and health back to its original design; reduces inflammation flare-ups; aligning your life with heaven's purpose; in need of healing and helping hands.

CLOWN: Having fun; "clowning around"; foolish jesting; goofing off; carnal nature; hiding true identity in comedy and fun; people-pleaser; demons disguised. See Eph 5:4.

CORPSE: Spiritually dead in gifts; shut off the flow of the Holy Spirit.

COUNSELOR: Christ; blessings in wise counsel; plans succeed with many advisors; professional advice; where there is no counsel, people will fall. See Is 9:6, Pro 12:15, 1:14, 15:22.

CUSTODIAN/JANITOR: Clean up others' messes; mother dreaming of responsibilities; trusted to maintain cleanliness and order in the house (could be Church). See 1 Chr 9:17–26.

DAUGHTER: Literal daughter; spiritual responsibility; mentoring a younger one ("like mother, like daughter"); immature in gifts but growing.

DEAD RELATIVE: Working through grieving process; encouragement to carry out family calling and use of gifts; bring wisdom.

DOCTOR: Healing minister; Jesus; restoration/repair; literal doctor.

DRIVER: Person in control; if no license–no authority to be in control; if reckless–someone taking charge who could hurt others; driving in reverse–going backward in your calling or career.

EX: Old love; old lifestyle; going back to something you were once committed to in the past; literal; past failure; issues with the past (need to forgive, holding on to past, grudge).

FACELESS PERSON: Angel, Holy Spirit, demon; someone whose identity is hidden or unimportant.

FAMILY: Church family; natural family and relatives; friends like family; generational blessings or curses.

FARMER: Christ; minister, laborer in the field (plow the ground); sower of seeds; those who spread the gospel or teach the Word (apostle, prophet, evangelist, pastor, or teacher); missions; Christians.

FATHER: God; authority; someone like a father to you; spiritual father; protector; provider; corrects; leads; loves; literal father; the foolish reject father's discipline; satan, the father of lies. See Rom 4:6, Pro 3:11, 13:24, 15:5, 20:7, Matt 7:9–11.

FIREMAN: Jesus (Savior and Rescuer from the fire); evangelist; angel; someone who puts out fires (i.e., gossip).

FOREIGNER: Unbeliever; calling to minister to a particular group; unknown; (do not oppress the foreigner or stranger). See Lev 19:34, Zech 17:10.

GARDENER: God; tending to growth and character; weeding out what is not needed. See also *Farmer*.

GRANDCHILD: New generation; crown to the aged; your legacy; spiritual blessings passed down; have influence over; literal grandchild. See Pro 17:6.

GRANDPARENT: Spiritual heritage; generational blessings or curses passed down (what runs through the family line). See Num 14:18.

HUSBAND: Jesus; covenant relationship (commitment may be membership or contracts); Church; lifelong project; literal husband.

INDIAN: Someone there first; connected to nature; spiritual (positive or negative); warrior.

JUDGE: God; justice; "hearing" your petition; righteous judgment.

MECHANIC: Jesus; ministers; someone helping to repair things in life.

MOTHER: Church; Holy Spirit; one like a mother; nurturer and protector; show her honor and live long; literal mother. See Eph 6:2.

NEIGHBOR: Brother or sister in Christ; neighboring church or ministry; connection in your ministry or job; literal neighbor; sharing common concerns, coworker.

OLD LOVE: Returning to old ways; something you let go of that you desire again; trying to fill a need with something from the past; returning to an old habit. See also *Ex.*

PIRATE: Criminal of the seas; attacks ships (ministries); takes by force; lawlessness.

POLICE: Authority; legalism; angel; helper/rescuer; "police the area"; encourage safety for people; if you get a ticket from a police officer, it indicates correction and discipline.

PROPHET: Prophetic ministry; God brings a word to you through a messenger; literal prophet. See Num 12:6.

RELATIVE: Family; bloodline; family issues; person placed in your life whom you did not choose.

SISTER: Sister in the Lord; literal; share similarities or similar circumstances; someone close like a sister.

SOLDIER: God's help sent to protect; spiritual warfare; time of opposition and war; we are soldiers in the Lord's army; reminder to put on our spiritual armor. See Eph 6:11, 2 Tim 2:3.

SON: Literal son; disciple; child of God; wordplay "sun"; carries family name; spiritual son; someone you are equipping.

STRANGER: Angel; demon; thief; helper; reminder to help those in need. See Gal 5:14, Heb 13:2.

TEAM: Group you are in fellowship with (family, church, work); unity. See Ps 133:1.

VAMPIRE: Sucks the blood and life out of you; a warning to avoid someone who is draining you; spirit of suicide; cutting; acts that draw blood; commanded not to drink blood. See Lev 17:12.

WIFE: Bride of Christ; covenant relationship; something you are committed to (ministry, career, person); literal wife; Israel.

UNKNOWN MAN OR WOMAN: Someone you know who reminds you of a man or woman; yourself.

YOUNG BOY OR GIRL: Young church; ministry in need of teaching/training, immature in gifts or experience; disciple; youth.

BODY PARTS

ACNE: Something irritating; gets under your skin; affects your image; seeing others' flaws; dietary/junk food warning; need for cleansing and care to save face. See Song of Sol 4:7.

ANKLES: Flexibility in your walk; connections; movement (or lack of); sore ankle—something hindering your walk; weak ankles–weak faith; sprained ankle–you need time to heal from something you stumbled into.

ARM: Strength; power; deliverance and redemption with God's outstretched arm; victory (raised arms); right arm—God's strength, deliverer; left arm—man's strength; to give weapons to someone ("arms"). See Ex 6:6, 17:11, Ps 89:13, Isa 62:8.

BACK: Past; backbone to stand up to something; strength to bear burdens; things behind you; areas you cannot see; someone who turns their back on you is ignoring you; someone "backing" you financially; someone who "has your back"; gossip ("backbiter"); criticism for taking a stand ("backlash"). See Jer 32:33, Gen 19:26, Luke 9:62.

BEARD: Maturity; covering; wisdom (especially if white); strength. See Lev 21:5.

BELLY: Holy Spirit in man ("out of your belly shall flow rivers of living water"); digest spiritual food/teachings; intuition ("gut feeling"); appearance of health; "belly of hell"; satisfaction from food or desire; the heart; Jonah in the belly of the whale; curse of the serpent. See Gen 3:14, Jon 1:17, 2:2, Jn 7:38, Phil 3:19, Tit 1:12, Rom 16:18, Pro 18:18, 20:27, 22:18, 26:22.

BONES: Structural support in your life; strength; death (can these bones live?: dead men's bones); spirit; health; people of Israel ("dry bones"); pleasant words are health to bones. See Matt 23:27, Ez 37:3&11, Pro 16:24.

BREAST: Nurture; comfort the spiritually immature; keeping "abreast" of matters; nourishment; mothering; lust.

CALVES: Support your walk; strength.

CHEEK: Beauty; displays countenance/emotions (smile, frown, blush); friendship kiss or greeting; assault/slap; forgiveness ("turn the other cheek"); cheeky (wisecrack). See Song of Sol 5:13, Matt 5:39, Rom 16:16.

CHIN: Determination; perseverance; "stick your chin out"; encouragement (chin up); ego.

EAR: Incline your ear for spiritual hearing; hearers of the Word; listen to instruction and wisdom; prophetic; "I'm all ears" (undivided attention); "play it by ear" (no planning or instruction); "itching ears" (find doctrine that feels good). See Is 55:3, 2 Tim 4:3.

ELBOW: Humility; support the work of your hands; need some elbow room; "elbow grease" (hard work); funny bone.

EYES: Vision; window to the soul; spiritual sight versus natural; lust of the eyes; bulging or overly dilated eyes–trying to see more than you are gifted to see; blind eyes–not being able to see in the spirit; the "ayes" have it.

FACE: Self-image; reflects one's heart; countenance reflects emotion (i.e., joy, sorrow, depression, confidence); something you are "facing"; "save face."

FEET: Your walk in life; messenger; satan under your feet; walk by faith; gospel of peace; Word of God or lack of it; the Word is a lamp for your feet; being "walked on" (taken advantage of); "getting back on your feet"; "get your feet wet" (try something new); "cold feet" (hesitate); "put your foot in your mouth" (say something offensive); "get your foot in the door" (opportunity); bare feet (unprepared or on holy ground). See Ex 3:5, Rom 10:15, 16:20, 2 Cor 5:7, Ps 119:105.

FINGERS: Fivefold ministry gifts (thumb/ apostle, index/ prophet, middle/ evangelist; ring/ pastor, pinkie/ teacher); work of your hands; covenant marriage ring; feelings; pointing accusations.

FOREHEAD: Mind; beliefs; revelation; mark of the beast on forehead or hand. See Rev 13:16.

HAIR, BALD: Lacking a spiritual covering; losing strength; aging; lacking wisdom; shaven head indicates putting away sinfulness or past traditions. See Num 8:7, Mic 1:16, Jud 16:19.

HAIR: Covering; wisdom; strength; a woman's glory is her long hair; men's rebellion with long hair; past; culture; style of ministry; God know the number of hairs on your head; messy hair—confusion. See 1 Cor 11:15, Luke 12:7.

HAIRCUT: Breaking religious tradition; cutting off wisdom; loss of strength (Samson); breaking away from cultural norms. See Jud 16:19.

HAND: Works; worship; agreement ("shake on it"); getting a handle on things; getting out of hand or control; strength; anointing; lend a "helping hand"; laying on of hands/impartation; ministry work; bless with your hands; to offer. Left hand–inherited; if you are left hand–dominant, what is easy for you may require more faith for others; what you were born to do and gifted with. Right hand—gifts of faith; "right-hand man"; the right way or choice; oath; promise; if you are right hand–dominant, then what you do well you do naturally; to move in your gifts; extend the right hand of fellowship. Washing hands–sanctification, washing hands from a situation you do not want to be involved in; if compulsive then sign of guilt. See Lev 9:22, 1 Tim 2:8, 4:14, Ps 90:17, 134:2.

HEAD: Authority; leader; head knowledge versus spiritual knowledge.

HEEL: Weakness (Achilles' heel); can cause a fall; person who treats others unfairly ("a heel"); "heal." See Gen 3:15.

HIP: Support; reproduce; stubborn (Jacob's hip socket was touched); passion. See Gen 32:25.

KNEES: prayer; reverence; submission ("every knee shall bow"); humility; worship; strength. See Rom 14:11, Eph 3:14, Job 4:4.

LEGS: Pillar of support; strength; mobility; your walk; time (first leg, second leg, etc.).

LIPS: Speech; praise (fruit of your lips); keep the vows voluntarily vowed from your own lips; kiss (greeting, passion); doctrine; polished speech with lip gloss; color speech with lipstick; protect speech with chapstick; lip service (say one thing but do another). See Deut 23:23, Is 29:13, Ps 51:15, 63:3, Mal 2:6-7, Heb 13:15.

MOUTH: Words; what you communicate to others; out of your mouth are words from your heart; testimony; life and death are in the power of the tongue; encouraging or gossip; intimacy of a kiss; speak blessings or curses, speak truth or lies; sing praises or condemnation; "mouthing off"; stink bugs in mouth–words that stink and offend; bees in mouth–words that sting. See Matt 15:18, Pro 6:23, 18:21, Ps 27:1.

NECK: Will; beauty; honor (kings place gold around neck); strength; grace; vulnerability; ability to see in all directions; stiff-necked (stubborn); connects the head and the heart; if injured then a disconnect between mind and spirit; yoke (burden) on neck; "pain in the neck." See Deut 28:48, Jer 17:33, Pro 1:9, 3:22, Ex 32:9, Acts 7:51.

NOSE: Discernment; sensing situations or the environment; nosey; "knows;" sniffs out; red nose—possible addictions.

SHOULDER: Strength; leadership; able to shoulder a burden or weight; ruler, government; in the flesh trying to carry what you are not equipped to carry. See Luke 12:48, Is 9:6, Ps 81:6.

SIDE: Vulnerability; friendship; new relationship.

STOMACH: See *Belly*.

TEETH: Ability to chew on/process information; bite into an idea or concept; eye teeth–ability to understand what is seen; wisdom teeth–ability to make wise decisions; loss of teeth-losing wisdom in an area of life; loss of front teeth affects your image; incisors–ability to be decisive and cut through things with understanding; false teeth–man's wisdom; incorrectly processing ideas; braces—season of aligning and training; losing baby teeth indicates maturing to stronger teaching. See Ps 119:9, Zech 9:7-8.

THIGH: Oath or promise (hand under thigh); faith; strength; reproduction. See Gen 24:2.

TOES: Important for traction and balance in walking and running.

TONGUE: Words; health and life; taste. See Pro 12:18, 18:21, Ps 34:8. See also *Mouth.*

CLOTHING & WEARABLE ITEMS

APRON: Service to others.

ARMOR: God's protection; helmet — mind and thoughts; breastplate — heart and righteousness; feet — walk and preparedness; belt — truth; sword — Word of God; shield — faith; preparing for spiritual warfare. See Eph 6:11.

BACKPACK: Carrying essentials; burden; going to school; training; hiking.

BADGE: Authority.

BAND-AID: Temporary fix.

BANDAGE: Healing and restoration for wounded. See Is 1:6.

BASKET: Blessings; first-fruits offering; provision. See Deut 28:5, 26:2.

BELT: Truth; walk in truth (armor of God); hold your act together; you've got it "under your belt" (completed and taken care of).

BIKINI: Unhindered; going against church norms; uncovered; carnal nature.

BLINDFOLD: In the dark about something; truth is being withheld from you; blinded by your own beliefs rather than understanding God's truth. See Rev 3:17, 1 Jn 2:11.

BOOTS: Ability to trudge through difficult circumstances; missions; something you are called to do, such as a job; fieldwork; protection; work; fashion; "give someone the boot" (kick them out of a job, relationship, home, etc.).

BOXING GLOVES: Preparing to fight something; knocking it out (e.g., sickness, opposition); self-defense; praying for another who needs you to fight for them; being prepared with the Word of Truth to aim at your opponent. See 1 Cor 9:26.

BRA: Support; covering; intimacy.

BRIDAL GOWN: See *Wedding Dress*.

CLOTHES: Anointing; authority; job; attitude; culture; time period; calling/purpose; preparation; protection.

COAT: Mantle; authority; protection from cold; calling/anointing; cover another; double portion (Elijah); honor/favor (Joseph); hidden agenda; self-righteous. See Gen 37:3, 2 King 2:13.

CROWN: Royalty; authority; power. See 1 Pet 5:4, 2 Tim 4:8, Jam 1:12, Rev 14:14.

CULTURAL CLOTHES: Mission call to a particular nation; cultural issues; prayer for the country whose people wear that type of clothes.

EARRINGS: Spiritual hearing; paying attention; adornment; offering; gift; culture; bond servant. See Num 31:50, Ez 16:12.

GLASSES: Vision enhancement; "I can see clearly now"; issues of nearsightedness or farsightedness.

HAT: Protect your thoughts; covering; undercover.

JEANS: Durable; casual; genetics (genes/jeans); generational; Levi's/Levite (consecrated for the Lord's service).

LINGERIE: Time for comfort and relaxation; a matter of revealing too much or too little. See also *Underwear*.

LIPSTICK: Draw attention to your words; enhance beauty; seductress; color used can inform about tone of words. See Pro 5:3.

LOCKET: Commitment; holding on to a memory; gift; spiritual gift you have chosen to walk in that is apparent to others; devotion to a person or group; generational gift from a grandmother or mother passed to you; close to your heart.

MASK: Hiding true identity; difficulty facing things; projects a false image to others; theater; to hide.

NAKED: Vulnerable; unprepared; exposing who you really are (can be good); from waist down—reproductive; top half exposed—nurturing but not reproductive; if sexy, then drawing attention to self negatively.

NAME TAG: Identity; allows others to know who you are; a label or identity within a certain group that defines one of your roles; association with a group getting acquainted with you.

NECKLACE: Adornment for the neck (strength and authority); graceful; gift for speaking or singing; deceiving bondage.

OVERALLS: Labor; hard time; farming; country.

PANTS: What you are walking in or called to do; head of the home ("who wears the pants in the family").

PURSE: Carries your identity, finances (gained or lost); looking for identity and purpose.

RING: Covenant; promise; adornment; social status; promise; king's signet seal; authority; "full circle."

SHIRT: Your covering or mantle; displaying your gifts.

SHOES: Feet prepared for your calling or what you walk in (ministry, job, mission, life); preparation; trying to live up to expectations of your predecessor ("those are big shoes to fill"); barefoot—unprepared to walk in your calling, holy ground; too small shoes—walking in a position you have outgrown; big shoes—a big position you are called to, or trying to walk in a position you have not grown into or developed into yet; house shoes—comfortable in your walk (maybe too comfortable?) but have limited mobility; clown shoes—not taking your position seriously or clowning around; red slippers—a desire to return home or to go back, wisdom; high heels—elevated position, dressed for success, formal, professional, self–elevation; platform shoes creating your own platform, pride; tennis shoes—prepared to run; unmatched shoes—unequally yoked in your walk. See Ex 3:5, Ezek 16:10, Eph 6:15.

SHORTS: Leisure; casual approach to your work; not walking in the fullness of your calling (cut off); walk in the Lord with some exposure; leisurely approach to your walk; not prepared.

SWIMWEAR: Ready to jump into the things of the Spirit.

UNDERWEAR: Protective covering; vulnerability; unprepared; intimacy; in secret; private issues. See also *Lingerie*.

VEIL: Covering; concealed; separation; pending covenant of marriage.

WATCH: Time; prayer and intercession; "watchman on the wall"; a call to watch and observe. See Is 62:6.

WEDDING DRESS: Bride of Christ; intimacy; preparation for covenant marriage; Church making herself ready.

WIG: False or wrong thinking; false or fake covering.

PLACES

AIRPORT: Making connections; waiting for ministry or career to take off; about to go higher; the church who sends out many.

ALLEY: Off the main path; transition; unprotected area; danger; often a dead end; dark and lonely; fear; depression; hopelessness.

ALTAR: Place of repentance, prayer, and worship; make sacrifices in your life; wordplay for alter your ways for God's higher ways.

AMPHITHEATER: Something is magnified as it plays out; something is going to be amplified or played out in the open.

AMUSEMENT PARK: Thrills; folly; variety.

ANTARCTICA: Cold; remote; feeling isolated from others.

APARTMENT: Temporary life situation; others are sharing in common circumstances (financial, church, health).

ARMORY: Preparation for military action; storage of weapons.

ATTIC: Times past; stored memories; the mind; often needs to be uncluttered from the past; treasures/gifts neglected; history; inherited generational issues (good or bad); upper room.

BACKSTAGE: Working behind the scenes; humility; out of the spotlight.

BAKERY: Providing spiritual life to others; delivers the Word of God; moneymaker ("dough").

BALLROOM: Formal occasion; celebration; bridegroom and bride dance; fun.

BANK: Financial storehouse; favor; usury; heavenly account; provision; dealing with money; institution of man; you can "bank" on it; the church where you sow tithes and offerings. See Matt 6:20, Luke 19:23, Jn 2:15.

BANQUET: Abundance; celebration; Marriage Supper of the Lamb; fellowship; celebration. See Song of Sol 2:4, 1 Cor 10:21.

BAR: Social meeting place with "spirits" (alcohol). See 1 Cor 6:10.

BARBERSHOP: Cut off wisdom; cut off old way of thinking, traditions, or habits; remove old covenants or false religious ideas and sin; new style of ministry or job; change your image. See Jud 17:17, Rom 12:2.

BARN: Place of storage; harvest; greed; storehouse of provision and blessings; may not be time to be released; accumulating; wealth; church. See Matt 13:30, Pro 14:4, Luke 12:18–21.

BASEMENT: Foundational issues or beliefs; hidden below the surface; hidden agendas; if cracked, there is too much weight or pressure; core beliefs (strong or weak); primary issues. See Jer 38:6.

BATHROOM: Place for cleansing spiritual toxins from life; preparation; polish your act; pamper; if there are no doors, then private issues transparent to others or concern for how others see you; public bathroom could be involvement in others' messes, uncomfortable place for relief, or an uncomfortable private matter; filthy home bathroom–could be dealing with so many messes in your family that it affects your own needs (can be a church or dealing with other people's problems); can't find bathroom could indicate an inability to find a place of refreshing and processing; constipation could indicate holding in toxic emotions. See Is 1:16, Pro 17:14, 2 Sam 11:2, 4.

BEACH, SEASHORE: Time with God; where humanity meets the deep things of God; recreation; soaking in the Son/sun; refreshing spiritually and mentally; lost in time ("sands of time"); mission-minded; facing something uncertain in life.

BEAUTY SHOP, SALON: Grooming for ministry; finding your style; preparation; vanity. See Pro 31:30, Hos 10:5, Ps 29:2, 1 Cor 11:15. See also *Barbershop*.

BED: Rest; intimacy; people in bed with you, such as a family (sharing the same issues; where you begin and end each day); a place for dreams and visions. See Ps 4:4, 139:8, Is 28:18–20, Heb 13:4, Jam 4:4.

BEDROOM: Rest; peace; intimacy; privacy, consider context:your current bedroom, things affecting you now; your childhood bedroom–disturbances from past issues still needing prayer.

BILLBOARD: Big message; trying to get your attention; bills; finances.

BRIDGE: Transition; crossing over to something new; mediator between God and man is the cross; going over; linking and networking; stuck on a bridge or living on the bridge–something is holding you back or fear of moving forward; falling or collapsing bridge—unstable direction, timing issue, or fear of failure.

BUILDING: Church; business; self-condition. Number of floors could inform about level.

CABIN: Time alone; solitary place; peace.

CAFETERIA: Church; place for serving many people spiritual food; community; variety. See Matt 25:35, Ps 19:9–10, Jn 6:27, 48, 63, 1 Cor 3:1–2, Heb 5:14.

CAMP: Gather troops; temporary dwelling; fellowship; under an open heaven; simplify. See Deut 23:14.

CASTLE: Fortress; ancient strongholds; unchanging; city of God; church. See 2 Chr 17:12.

CAVE: Solitary place; hiding; everything stripped away to concentrate on God; hiding from the world and calling; isolation; dwelling place; tomb. See 1 King 18:4.

CEMETERY: Burying the past; reminder of temporal life; new life in Christ; death.

CHURCH: Bride of Christ; organization of believers; teaching and preaching the gospel of Jesus; equipping center to train believers for the harvest field.

CLASSROOM: Education and learning; equipping center; place of testing. See 2 Tim 2:15.

CLIFF: High place requiring faith and skill; "cliffhanger"; suspense; on edge.

CLOSET: Hidden; place of prayer; stores clothes and shoes for what we are called to walk in; hiding something; "skeletons in the closet."

COFFIN: Death; the end of something (e.g., job, school, relationship); dealing with grief; timing has ended; "driving the final nail in the coffin" means something that was already failing has finally ended.

CORRAL: Limitations; hedge.

COUNTRY STORE: Get the basics; simple times.

COURT: Going through a trial; need for justice; plead your case; innocent or guilty judgment; enemy is accuser of the brethren/Jesus paid the penalty for us. See Is 43:25.

COURTHOUSE: Going through a trial. See also *Court.*

CROSSROAD: Major decision affecting the path of your life.

CRUISE SHIP: Church; workplace; relaxing; pleasure; diversion from responsibility.

DESERT: Spiritually dry place; barren and unproductive; time of testing in a wilderness experience. See Num 14:26–30.

DINING ROOM: Communion and fellowship; place of spiritual nourishment/the Word.

DOORWAY: Threshold; place of opportunity; access. See Jn 10:7, Col 4:3, Ps 141:3.

ELEVATOR: Going through emotional ups and downs; going up or down in favor and anointing.

FACTORY: Mass-production center; work or church; repetitive; organizational teamwork; reproduction. See Luke 2:49, Rom 12:11, Pro 31:13, 1 Thes 2:9, Acts 20:35.

FIELD: World; harvest; growth potential; gospel to the mission field; work in the field; field of study; out in left field (ideas that are way off).

FOUNDATION: Strength or weakness of your support system; cracked—problem in the house or church; basic foundational beliefs.

FUNERAL: Death; end of something close to you; if it is your funeral—death of fleshly desires, habits, or lifestyle.

GARAGE: Storage; keeps your ministry secure and rested; parked and not going anywhere.

GARDEN: Heart; cultivating and tending your spiritual growth; God's blessings; fruit of your spirit; time to blossom; ministry labor for the harvest; sowing and reaping; fragrance of the Lord. See Gen 2:8.

GAS STATION: Place to refresh and refuel to power you for further work; fresh refill of spiritual encouragement.

GYMNASIUM: Local impact ministry; exercise faith and discipline; youth-oriented ministry.

HALLWAY: Transition period; walk it out without a lot of options.

HIGH RISE: High spiritual calling; promotion; revelatory gift (see from a higher perspective); luxury living.

HIGHWAY: Fast-paced spiritual journey; life in the fast lane; journey.

HOSPITAL: Healing; the Church; restoration of ministries, hearts, and brokenness; physical; ministry of healing.

HOTEL: Temporary place or situation; get touched and move on; in the midst of change; will cost something; short-lived.

HOUSE: You or your life; family or a group; "where your heart is"; the Church; the condition you are in or the group (spiritually).

ICU: Intensive critical care needed to save souls; urgent and critical situation.

ICY ROAD: Slippery path; caution. See Ps 73:18, Jer 23:12.

IGLOO: Cold emotions in a home; icy, slippery, or cold situation.

JACUZZI: Personal move of the Spirit.

JAIL: Bondage; spiritual, emotional, or physical limited mobility; captivity; under the law; paying for crime/sin.

JUNGLE: Survival and perseverance in your field of work or study; "It's a jungle out there"; brutally competitive; uncivilized.

KITCHEN: The heart; a place for preparing spiritual food or teaching; where the spiritually hungry gather; "if you can't take the heat, get out of the kitchen."

LAKE: Water of the Holy Spirit; sphere of influence; atmosphere that surrounds your life.

LIBRARY: Exploration of knowledge; borrow information at no expense; books of remembrance; place of gathering facts; unable to talk; a place of whispers.

LIGHTHOUSE: Guidance in dark or stormy times; spiritual truth; decisions needing clarity; keep your focus on God to lead you home. See Ps 27:1, Pro 6:23.

LIVING ROOM: Where you/your family lives and interacts; place of fellowship.

LOCKER ROOM: Preparing to get in the game; temporary storage.

MALL: Marketplace; many options available; need special provisions for an upcoming situation (specialty shops); materialism; outreach to those looking for something; get what you need in one place but will cost you.

MAZE: The Lord helping you out of a confusing time; need direction left or right; caught in a "rat race."

MOBILE HOME: Temporary dwelling; financial strain; may mean you need to move on; could indicate your literal home. See also *Trailer.*

MOON: The Bride/Church reflects the sun; cycles and seasons; blood moon. See Gen 1:16, Is 30:26, Acts 2.

MOUNTAIN: Elevated place of visitation; vision for seeing; obstacles; kingdoms. See Rev 6:14, Ps 18:33, Song of Sol 1:7.

MOVIE THEATER: Vision; seeing the "big picture"; life drama; scenes playing out; spectator in life; performance/ entertainment-minded church; something dramatic coming; entertainment from actors/pretense.

MUSEUM: Something is showcased but untouchable; preserved past.

NEIGHBORHOOD: Community sharing the same issues.

NURSERY: Caring for what God has birthed in the spirit; new and vulnerable ministries, people, or jobs needing lots of care; getting ready to birth something.

OFFICE: Place where you use your skills and gifts; work; administrative; what you are called to do; office in the Body of Christ (e.g., prophet or apostle) working at something; job-related issues.

OUTDOORS: Open heaven; getting things out in the open; stepping out of comfort zone.

PALACE: Mansion; royalty; lush; lifestyle; blessing of the Lord.

PARK: Playful; picnics; celebrations of friends and family; relaxing; diversion from work; "parked" or stalled; in need of motivation.

PIT: Hell; trap; grave.

PLATFORM: Something that is built to support your work and target an audience; elevated.

POOL: Holy Spirit; spiritual life (holy or unholy).

PORCH: Front porch—future, vision; back porch—past, looking back, history; side porch—approaching things your way as opposed to following the standard procedures.

PORT: Calling to influence that region ("port of call"); a place to stop for supplies.

PRISON: See also *Jail.*

RESTAURANT: Place of teaching and service for the spiritually hungry (could be the Church); looking for options in your life; provides choices to accommodate many spiritual levels (milk versus meat of the Word); looking for something to satisfy; cost involved; others will serve you; potential to serve many people at once.

ROAD: Spiritual journey; the paths you choose to follow.

ROLLER RINK: Going in circles; recreation.

ROOF: Spiritual covering; the mind; protection and shield.

SCHOOL YARD: Freedom from training is coming.

SCHOOL: Learning; training; teaching; old school- the old way; educational level; the grade informs about the level of learning; season of learning; place of testing; equipping; something God wants to teach you; something you did not learn the first time, especially if it's your old school; new school learning something new or from a different perspective; fear of failure; elementary—going back to the basics; middle school—transition between immature and the mature; high school and college—advancement in higher learning and promotion.

SHACK: Poverty; tough times; poor spiritual, emotional, or physical condition and neglect.

SPACE: Satellite communications; global impact; heavenly sphere; "spacy" person.

STADIUM: Huge impact; impacts many people.

STAGE: Public recognition; you are being observed and in the spotlight; influence; a platform to speak or act; where things are played out; acting and entertaining; "setting the stage"; preparing to make things happen.

STAIRWAY: Going up or down in your journey; promotion; transition; highs and lows; taking a step at a time; step by step; going up to a higher spiritual place or coming down to daily life.

SWAMP: Stuck; "swamped"; overwhelmed; nasty environment. See also *Swamp* in Weather and Earth Conditions.

TENT: Temporal; fleshly body; impact large or small; evangelism (tent revival); camping out versus dealing with something; temporary situation; communion with God.

TREEHOUSE: Simple hidden place in God; childlike faith; residence among leaders.

TUNNEL: Birthing transition; passage to a new place hidden in God; coming out of an old place.

UPSTAIRS: Higher place of vision; upper room; anointing; could be thoughts/mind.

VINEYARD: Spiritual condition fruitful or overgrown; Israel; new wine.

WAREHOUSE: Heaven's provision and storage; resources available to you; stored-up things to get off the shelf (e.g., creative ideas, provision, blessings).

WORK ZONE: Change; develop new ideas; spiritual work; construction of something new.

YARD: Part of your life on display; back yard is more private for family gatherings and events; front yard is more public.

ZOO: Captives of the wild; "what a zoo"; it's wild, confusing, disorderly.

WEATHER &
EARTH CONDITIONS

AUTUMN: Fall harvest; preparation for winter.

BAROMETER: Under pressure; pressure; stress in your environment; predicts changes that are coming.

BLIZZARD: White-out; blinding your vision; cold storm coming; grounded; immobilizing.

BLUE SKY: Open heaven; revelation.

CLOUDS: Covering; protection; witnesses; signs in the heavens above; warning of a storm coming (spiritual or literal); dark clouds—from the enemy, an attack on the mind, judgment, depression, grief, confusion. See Ps 18:11.

CREEK: Small stream or influence; place where children learn.

DEW: Blessing from the Lord; moisture to cover and refresh the land; quickly disappears. See Gen 27:28, Hos 13:3.

DROUGHT: Experiencing a spiritually dry time; need for spiritual refreshing; trials seem harsh and life is routine; just getting through it. See Is 58:11, Ps 32:4.

EARTHQUAKE: Life is about to be shaken; shift in foundational beliefs; warning; judgment; literal. See Num 16:32–34, 1 Sam 14:15, Hag 2:6–7, Acts 16:26.

FLOOD: Judgment, as in the days of Noah; literal disaster; if from the Lord—revival, a great outpouring of the Spirit, cleansing, going deeper in the things of God; if flooding your house—the move will be personal; if from the enemy—muddy, destructive force bringing ruin and loss, creates circumstances that keep you from progressing. See Luke 17:27.

FOG: Unclear time; walk by faith not by sight; confusion; clouded judgment.

FROST: Blessings frozen in time; damages your fruit in frigid conditions; temporary.

HAIL: Judgment; cold, hard conditions; curse. See Rev 16:21.

HEAT WAVE: Oppression; scorching; anger of the Lord; south wind; time of testing; scorching time; "turn up the heat." See Matt 20:12, Ex 11:8, Jud 2:14, Is 25:5.

HIGH TIDE: Shifting of opinions of the world; timing; gravitational or unseen pull; reaching high levels; blessings coming in; people coming to salvation.

HUMID: Smothering; hope and teaching coming.

HURRICANE: Trial; judgment; opposition; destructive winds of change.

ICE: Inactive; coldhearted; frozen assets or a situation on hold; put something on delay; cold person; winter season; stopping flow of the Holy Spirt; spiritually cold church; frozen in time; dangerous/slippery; thin ice is risky.

ICEBERG: Only seeing the tip of the problem (i.e., "tip of the iceberg"); deeper issues unseen; hidden mass under the surface.

LAKE: Your spiritual life.

LIGHTNING: Power released; judgment; fall of satan; flashes of inspiration. See Job 36:32.

NIGHT: Hidden; uncertain; unrevealed; dark night of the soul (i.e., depression); children of the night in sin; increased crime; nightwatch prayer. See 1 Thes 5:5, Jn 8:12.

OCEAN: Humanity; mysterious; uncertain; unlimited opportunities; overseas; influence over many people; missions; deep things of God; the Word.

POND: Small group or individual spiritual influence; "big fish in a small pond."

QUICKSAND: Stuck; "in over your head"; your struggles against it make it worse; on a loose foundation; being overwhelmed; hopeless situation; sinking in an area of life or into depression; requires assistance to get you out.

RAIN: Spiritual outpouring; blessings; renewal; rains on just and unjust; cleansing; brings growth.

RAINBOW: Covenant; reminder of God's promises; gay and lesbian symbol; promises of God displayed in the sky. See Gen 9:13.

RIVER: Move of God; several streams (other groups) join in unified purpose; being in transition when moving from one side to the other; lazy river (i.e., not using your gifts).

SMOKE: Presence of God; "where there is smoke, there's fire;" offensive as "smoke to the eyes." See Is 6:3–4, Pro 10:26.

SNOW: Blanket of white; purity; grace; righteousness; cold; stuck ("snowed in"); "pure as the driven snow"; heavy workload ("snowed under"). See Is 55:10–11.

SPRING: Time of planting; waking up from winter to a new season of life blooming.

SUMMER: Time of growth; fruitful; work by the sweat of the brow; "turn up the heat."

SWAMP: No move of the Spirit; stagnant; overgrown. See also *Swamp* in Places.

THUNDER: God's voice; warnings; judgment; argument. See Job 37:4–5.

TORNADO: Turbulent environment that can pull you into circumstances that will twist things around and be difficult; can be judgment from the Lord; if from the enemy will leave damage and chaos behind; if from the Lord (often white) will cause a cleanup and a positive outcome when it's all over; could be a call to get rid of dead things in your life before God does it for you; destructive winds of change. See Hos 8:7. See also *Whirlwind*.

TSUNAMI: Foundational shift below the surface with broad national consequences (governmental decisions, banking decisions, global impact); warning of coming crises with huge impact; on the positive side it could be a sudden move of God pouring out on the land; waves of revival coming; out of man's hands.

VOLCANO: Erupting emotions that boil within; judgment.

WAVES: Move of God's Spirit that comes in waves and recedes; repeating action; exciting and fun; could be judgment to the unprepared Church.

WHIRLPOOL: Two opposing streams converge into a vortex that can pull you under; chaos; swirling emotions or thoughts; gossip going around that will pull you in.

WHIRLWIND: Powerful vortex funnel forming over the earth; gossip going around that will pull you in; a powerful move of God's Spirit. See 2 King 2:11. See also *Tornado*.

WIND: Holy Spirit; east wind—judgment; west wind—blessing; changes coming; "winds of change"; the voice of God.

WINTER: Cold season of rest and planning; seemingly dead time.

TRANSPORTATION &
MEANS OF MOVEMENT

18-WHEELER: Huge influence to bring blessings or judgment. See also *Semitruck*.

AIRPLANE: Corporation, organization, or ministry (size depends on size of plane); flying high in your calling; taking off in ministry or business; moving to new spiritual heights; national or international calling; going beyond your boundaries; making connections; something up in the air (hasn't landed yet). See also *Jet*.

AMBULANCE: Administer urgent care; healing ministry; transitional care that treats then connects people according to their more specific needs.

ARK: God's protection for overwhelming floods or storms in life.

ARMY TANK: Power behind the scenes; spiritual warfare; heavily armored protection/prayer.

BACKHOE: Time to build; renovation or new project; timing; digging into something good or bad; going deeper.

BATTLESHIP: Church or ministry involved in spiritual warfare; rescue mission; war "overseas"; protector. See also *Ship*.

BICYCLE: Individual work; local influence requiring effort; growing in God. See Gal 5:4, 19.

BLIMP: Puffed up; pride; showy; no internal structure.

BOAT: Individual, church, or ministry; on a mission to save souls; rescue boat—save souls or wounded people; riverboat—a move of the Spirit that carries many people along; speedboat—quick move of the Spirit, ministry that comes in powerfully and goes out quickly; rowboat—getting started in ministry or job, requires a lot of effort, not equipped to take many others with you; sailboat—moved by the wind of the Holy Spirit, not man-powered; tugboat—helps minsters and leaders by giving a push to get going or assisting and towing them. See also *Ship.*

BUS: Ministry; large mission groups with common interests; double-decker—double anointing or favor; school bus— teaching ministry, youth; church bus—ministry outside the church. See 2 King 4:38, 2 Tim 2:2, Heb 11:9.

CANOE: Individual ministry requiring self-effort; good for small jobs and transitioning from one side to the other; going into hard-to-reach areas.

CAR: What you operate in; your life, work, or ministry; your drive/motivation; antique—restoration ministry or seeing potential in elderly ministry or a calling or job unfulfilled; armored—you or what you carry are protected, taking your ministry or job where protection is needed, insecure, overprotected; convertible—open heaven, free spirit, unprotected; former car—something you are still operating in from the past, an old system of operating, could represent a time period for something you need to resolve; limo—favor of God, celebrity, paying others a high price to take you places.

CHARIOT: A higher revelatory anointing; transcending time; biblical time period.

COVERED WAGON: Pioneering the way; difficult conditions; mission field. See also *Stagecoach.*

CRUISE SHIP: Church; fun; worldly; excess. *Titanic*—warning not to get on board a new big ministry because of unfavorable outcomes. See also *Ship* and *Boat.*

DELIVERY TRUCK: Provision from Christ to help meet the needs of others.

DUMP TRUCK: Construction in your life; dumping problems on others; carrying heavy loads; removing debris and filling in holes.

ELEVATOR: Easy access; going up or down in anointing or job; promotion or demotion. See also *Escalator.*

ESCALATOR: Going up or down a level in something in your life or work; effortless transition. See also *Elevator.*

FIRE TRUCK: Rescue mission; carries water of the Holy Spirit.

FLYING: Advancement in the spirit; rise above circumstances; calling to go to higher levels; learning to operate in the supernatural gifts.

FORKLIFT: Holy Spirit lifts you up; reaches where man cannot.

GO-CART: Recreational fun; going in circles; potential danger.

HANG GLIDER: Moved by the wind of the Spirit.

HELICOPTER: Small ministry that can maneuver in hard-to-reach places; rescue missions; can reach where people are stuck or wounded; flies below radar undetected by the enemy; job or ministry operating on short notice; hovering personality.

HORSEBACK: Individual power ministry.

HOT AIR BALLOON: Can rise above things; full of hot air; display.

JET: Flying high in the spirit; ministries or corporations; capacity to carry many others; influence; private jet—receiving instruction from the Lord, going alone on a special mission; intercession into the heavenlies. See also *Airplane.*

LADDER: Increase or decrease in anointing; climbing higher step by step; Jacob's ladder was a portal for angels to ascend and descend upon the earth. See Gen 28:12.

LAWN MOWER: Pruning; manicuring and beautifying the flesh; cutting down; means of repentance.

MOBILE HOME: Moving around in an aspect of your life; flexible; adaptable; unsettled; literal home.

MOTORCYCLE: Personal ministry in street and local community; free from religious constraints; can reach where other ministries cannot; powerful in groups; under an open heaven; can be rebellion; lack Christian covering; exposed to elements; fair weather ministry.

OCEAN LINER: Foreign (overseas); mission-minded church.

POGO STICK: Ups and downs; a lot of effort but going nowhere.

POLICE CAR: Authority, patrol; transports criminals; stops lawbreakers.

ROCKET: Far-reaching impact; being thrust higher in the things of the spirit or life; be careful to avoid burnout; launching into your destiny; powerful ministry taking off and going great distances.

ROLLER COASTER: Thrills of highs and lows that take you back where you began; fast track of ups and downs; thrill seeker; fear; you are not in control; exciting; "on an emotional roller coaster" (extreme highs and lows).

SEMITRUCK: Carrying partial blessings; more to come; not the whole story; big influence, depending on what it carries; operating in calling; capacity to transport goods to areas of need; marketplace ministry or job. See also *18-Wheeler.*

SHIP: Large mission-minded church, ministry, or business. See also *Battleship* and *Cruise Ship.*

SKATEBOARD: Personal ministry; community or neighborhood influence; quick words in passing and move on; hobby; skill.

SKATES: Individual ministry or job requiring legwork; fun and recreational; propels your walk; skating around an issue; requires balance; gliding over issues; ice-skating—"skating on thin ice," graceful, entertainment, operating on cutting edge. See Rom 9:28. See also *Roller Rink* in Places.

SKIING: Quick action; ability to quickly dodge issues; fast descent.

SPACESHIP: High spiritual encounter with God; a craft off-limits with God, going in unknown territory; getting off-track and out in space.

STAGECOACH: Rough ride, uncomfortable, old-fashioned way but will get you there. See also *Covered Wagon.*

STREETCAR: Street ministry; local church, ministry, or business; runs on track.

Terri Meredith

SUBMARINE: Moving undercover in deep things; mission unseen, such as intercessors; secret mission; working under the issues; below radar (undetected).

SUBWAY: Below the surface; making connections; "sub" way as oppose to "high" way; working under the issues.

SWIMMING: Being immersed in the things of the Spirit; refreshing; anointing; "keeping your head above water."

TAXI: Another ministry, person, or business that helps you get going, but comes with a cost and inconveniences.

TRACTOR: Pioneering ministry or business; preparing the fields for sowing and harvest of souls; ploughing up new ground.

TRAIN: Training and equipping groups; steady move of God or business; train cars could be departments, ministries, people, etc., comprising the entire entity; on track; "on the straight and narrow"; train wreck—disaster or failed program or ministry; derailed—off track.

TRUCK: Work; able to carry resources and supplies to areas of need; haul tools of trade.

UNICYCLE: Requires balance and skill to progress; unusual ministry; a ministry or business of one.

VAN: Influence to carry others in work or ministry.

WALKER: Used to provide assistance in your walk; infirmity.

WINGS: Freedom to fly or go higher. See *Flying.*

WOODEN RAFT: In survival mode; gaps in your life; stranded.

GENERAL

ABORTION: Termination of something; something precious lost; abort a plan or an opportunity; termination of something under development, a project, or a creative idea; literal abortion.

ACCIDENT: Warning of a potential mistake; someone's carelessness causing harm; warning to watch and pray.

AFFAIR: Spiritual adultery; putting others before God (idolatry); a new passion (i.e., job, school, hobby); spending most of your time on something other than God or spouse; literal affair.

AIRCONDITIONER: Conditions the atmosphere (as in praise/worship); cools things off.

AIRPLANE CRASH: Ending of a career or ministry; financial disaster.

ALARM: Wake-up call; warning; the time is now. See Joel 2:1.

ANCHOR: Prevents drifting; adds strength/weight; supports and keeps steady; hope. See Heb 6:19.

ANGELS: Heavenly messengers created by God; what they say or do should line up with the Word; if they indicate you should violate godly principles or laws, then they are not from God and should be considered an evil spirit. See Rev 14:6, Ps 91:11.

ANTIQUES: Old patterns and beliefs that are hard to let go of; passed down–generational inheritance (good or bad); loss of perceived usefulness.

APPLE: Teaching (fruit of the Spirit); fruit of your labor; health; temptation; apple of God's eye; prized possession; golden apple is wisdom; poison apple from the enemy is temptation that looks sweet but is forbidden. See Deut 32:10, Gen 3:6, Pro 25:11, Song of Sol 2:5.

AQUARIUM: Environment you live or work in; may feel you are being observed; confined.

ARMY: Trained for warfare; Christians taking a stand against darkness and sin; God's Special Forces; prayer warriors.

ARROWS: Children; intended to wound or kill; sharp words wounding deeply; launching a silent attack; poison arrows are poison words. See Job 6:2–4.

ARTIFICIAL INSEMINATION: A project or new endeavor initiated by man rather than God.

ASHES: Complete extermination; God gives beauty for ashes; restoration and hope. See Am 2:1.

AXE: Cutting away, as laying the axe to the root of sin and unproductiveness by the Word and prayer; tool to hew trees, which are symbolic of leaders. See Jer 51:20, Luke 3:9.

BABY, BIRTHING: Starting a new ministry or project; a gift coming requiring training; a premature birth is out of God's timing or happening sooner than expected.

BABY, NEGLECT: Not paying attention to your ministry gift; abandoning a project or gift you have care of; not making time for a new project or idea; a dead baby indicates the ending of something developing.

BAD BREATH: Offensive speech (may not be aware of it).

BAGS: Travel; carrying your troubles or excess baggage. See Ez 12:6, Is 10:28.

BAIT: Lure; evidence of a trap. See Am 3:5.

BAKING: Preparing the Word (spiritual food); provision. See 1 King 19:6. See also *Bread*.

BALM: Salve for healing; anointing for healing. See Jer 8:22.

BAND-AID: Temporary fix or cover-up.

BAND: Celebrate; joint effort; loud; the sound people carry for unified purpose; marching to the same tune. See Ps 68:25.

BANDAGE: Healing and restoration for wounded. See Is 1:6.

BANNER: Victory; His banner over you is love; victory flag. See Song of Sol 2:4, Ps 20:5.

BAPTISM: Commitment to be immersed and raised up to live for Him; spiritual renewal. See Matt 28, 16:20.

BARKING: Warning; intimidation; "his bark is louder than his bite." See Is 56:10.

BASEBALL: Get in the game of life; competition; waiting periods; hardball; fear of striking out.

BASKETBALL: Fast-moving conflicts ahead; stay alert and keep your focus; the ball may change hands many times before you score.

BEAMS: Infrastructure.

BESTIALITY: Abomination; lust; perversion; inordinate acts. See Lev 18:23, 1 Thes 4:3–5.

BINOCULARS: Seeing beyond your circumstances; vision for the future; insight; need to focus if blurry; getting a closer look at something.

BITING: "Biting off more than you can chew"; taking on too much; angry words that wound ("biting words").

BLANKET: Your covering (i.e., leader, head of household, boss); warmth and comfort; protection from a cold environment; security (i.e., security blanket); undercover of hidden issues; protection; love covers a multitude of sins; covers weaknesses and exposure; blanket protection is a mass covering, such as for congregations or groups of people; wearing a blanket like a chief could be authority. See 1 Pet 4:8.

BLIND: In the dark about something; spiritually blind regarding the things of God; blind leading the blind. See Matt 15:14, 1 Jn 2:11, 2 Pet 1:9.

BLOOD: Life; Jesus' sacrifice brings life; covenant; life is in the blood; bleeding you dry; drain financially; war; bloodline or generational issue passed down. See Heb 9:22, 1 Jn 1:7.

BOMB: Life-changing news (someone dropped a bomb); powerful event; major attack planned; potential for mass destruction; temper explosion (big blowup); end-time event.

BOOK OF LIFE: Important to note names written in it; warning to get right with God. See Rev 20:12, 21:27.

BOOMERANG: What you give out is going to come back to you (good or bad); a comeback. See Matt 5:7, Pro 26:27.

BOW: Shoots forth arrows (children); words of the wicked to harm the upright; spiritual warfare; spirit of truth; silent attack from the shadows. See Ps 11:2, Is 5:28, Rev 6:2.

BOXES: Hidden; boxed in (trapped by unscriptural religious ideas); storage (gifts not in use); moving; gifts and surprises; come out of hiding; exposing something (good or bad); unpack. See Luke 8:17.

BRAKES: Self-control; stop or slow down; the Lord preventing you from moving into trouble; a brake stuck indicates something holding you back; unable to stop on your own. See Acts 16:7, Num 22:32.

BREAD: Jesus; Word of Life; Scripture, wisdom of God; the Body of Christ; wisdom and truth of Jesus; leavened or unleavened to guard against false teaching; food in general; daily needs for survival. See Jn 6:51, Matt 4:4, Pro 92:5, Luke 11:3. See also *Baking*.

BRIDLE: Restraint; discipline; rebellion; bridle the tongue to control your words. See Jam 1:26, 3:3.

BRIEFCASE: Carry your work with you; on a special assignment that needs work; holding important information; your situation or case will be "brief"; calling to an executive-type position.

BROOM: Sweeping your spiritual house; repent for any wrongs; "make a clean sweep"; removing all unnecessary items at one time. See Jn 2:15, Gal 5:19–20.

BRUISE: Injury below the surface; Jesus was bruised for our iniquities; take a hit but will heal quickly.

BUFFET: Many choices.

BUTTER: Blessing; deceptive speech; "butter someone up"; manipulation; how you make a living (i.e., your bread and butter). See Ps 55:21.

CAKE: Celebrate; special occasion; "icing on the cake."

CALCULATOR: Counting the cost; seeing if things "add up"; calculating, as in discernment.

CALENDAR: Times; events; seasons. See Ecc 3:1.

CAMERA: Focusing in; capturing a moment in time; create memories; historian; instrument for gathering proof.

CANDLE: God's light; man's light; life; "snuffed out". See Pro 20:27.

CAR TROUBLE: Something missing or holding you back from moving forward.

CAR WASH: Cleansing and polishing your act; cleaning up something in your life, ministry, or career.

CAR WRECK: Warning; clash with other people; if totaled, then resolution will not come without the Lord's help; hitting other cars indicates careless decisions that will affect others; cars hitting yours is a warning to watch for others' reckless behavior affecting your life; out of control.

CEILINGS: Boundaries; limitations; "hit the ceiling" is the maximum return on investments; barrier blocking communication between you and God; the highest level that is perceived to be achievable.

CHAIR: Seat of authority or position; resting; your position; chairing a committee.

CHASING: Something you are running from or after in life; you have become a target for the enemy somehow; fear of being captured; something is following you that you are trying to escape, such as addiction; sin or your past following you; an issue you need to deal with in your life; a desire you are pursuing.

CHECK: Favor; gift; surprise; financial favor or obligation.

CHEW: Processing and breaking down new information; "chew on it" (meditate, think on it); "bite off more than you can chew."

CHOCOLATE: Crave affection and sweet words; treat yourself; feeds addictive behavior; gifts and surprises; have something sweet to offer others; feeding an emotion.

CHOKING: Blocking the breath of the Spirit; cutting your voice off; obstruction from something or someone that needs to be expelled; overwhelmed; bite off more than you can chew (an idea that is hard to swallow); quenching the Holy Spirit. See Job 33:4, Jn 20:22.

CIGARETTE: Puffed up (prideful); return to old habits; addiction; rebellion; risky behavior.

CIRCLE: Coming full circle; completed phase; going in circles; getting nowhere; wholeness; unity; covenant (ring).

COCONUT: A hard case but delightful when cracked; tropical.

COINS: Favor; changes coming; people; foreign coins are favor in that place. See also *Money*.

COMA: Not conscious of reality; life on hold.

CONSTRUCTION: Work in process; need of prayer to complete the work; a time of change and progress.

COOKING: Cooking up new ideas; spiritual teaching preparation; ideas on back burner (on hold), boiling, or simmering.

CORD: Strength (as in three-cord strand not easily broken); soul ties; tied to something. See Ecc 4:12.

COUCH: Comfortable place; peace; share with others; lazy (i.e., "couch potato"); couch an issue.

CREDIT CARD: Debt; what you enjoy today you will pay for tomorrow; the Lord extends favor/Christ paid the cost; lost credit card is lost credibility, favor, or trust.

CRYSTAL: Clarity and vision (crystal clear); valuable; New Age. See Job 28:18.

CUP: Life experience; sharing in blessings or hardships. See Jer 51:7.

CURB: Transition (to cross over, step into, or turn the corner in life), depending on direction and context; to mitigate or lessen (i.e., curb appetite).

CYMBAL: Praise and worship; something that can be painful to hear; warning or call to attention.

DAM: Holding back; blocking a move of God; harnessed power; damned/condemned; overwhelmed (good or bad); bursting dam could be opening the floodgates of blessings or curses. See Mark 16:16.

DART: Piercing words; curses; hitting the target; words that pierce; fiery darts from the enemy's accusations; an attack requiring the shield of faith. See Eph 6:16.

DASHBOARD: Navigation; monitors direction; tools to help you reach your destination; access to current and upcoming knowledge about a situation.

DEATH/DYING: The end of something (job, commitments, an issue, addiction); dying to self-will or old habits; dreamer dying –dying to self and living for Christ or a part of the dreamer dying; dreamer's child dying–something that was birthed, cared for, and/or nurtured (career or project) coming to an end; literal death; dead/unused spiritual gifts. See Heb 9:27.

DESK: Work; learning and study; writing.

DESSERT: Sweet ending; deceitful pleasures. See Pro 23:3.

DIAMONDS: Incredibly hard; valuable; expression of love and commitment (i.e., marriage/engagement); extreme pressure; can only be scratched by another diamond (by each other).

DIVING BOARD: A high place in life that springs you into your destiny; involves some risk; a challenge ahead of you; a place that may require a leap of faith; a position where you can see from above yet dive into the matter.

DIZZY: Going in circles; in need of spiritual equilibrium; need stability and balance; confusion.

DOOR: Christ ("I am the door"); opportunity; choices; Christ; front door–future; back door–past/previous experiences or family access; heavenly access (as in the foolish virgins parable); open door–open invitation (for good or evil); closed/locked door–protection, security, or denied access; glass doors–vision, what you walk through will be apparent to others, ability to see/prophetic; enter a side or back door–going against the system or unseen. See Col 4:3, Ps 141:3, Jn 10:1, 2, 7, 9, Matt 25:10.

DROWNING: Overwhelmed; hopelessness;in over your head; grief; depression; sorrow; overwhelming situation that feels like it has sucked the life out of you. See Matt 14:30.

DRUGS, STREET: Addiction; trap; temporary escape that replaces God; self-destruction; sin of witchcraft (the word *Pharmacia* is derived from the Greek "witchcraft"); a temptation or invitation into addiction. See 1 Sam 15:23.

DRY CLEANING: A spiritually dry atmosphere for cleansing; preparation for ministry or job; not the usual system; cleaning behind the scenes by a professional (i.e., counseling, pastoral care, small group therapy).

DUNG: Defilement; profane; offense; works of the flesh.

DYNAMITE: *Dunamis* power; big impact; miraculous works; highly explosive weapon; temper. See Matt 7:22, 11:21.

EAST: Christ will return from the East; sunrise; Eastern religious influence or ministry. See Matt 24:27.

EATING: Hungry for something; introducing information; diet and weight issues; what is eating at you.

EGG: New idea hatching; double yolks is double anointing; provision and hope; fertility; promises.

EMPTY: What is missing in life; need for salvation; depression; need for fulfillment.

ENGINE: Holy Spirit power working inside; heart; motivations or intentions (i.e., "driving force").

ESCAPE: Trying to flee a situation or bondage; seeking freedom from something; running rather than facing the issue.

EXAMINATION: Testing; not a time of learning and teaching but seeing whether you are ready.

EXPLOSION: Warning of sudden disaster; outburst of anger; big blowup.

FALLING: Losing control in an area of your life; losing support; backsliding; falling back into old ways or habits; regressing in job or life.

Terri Meredith

FAST FOOD: Quick access; "fills the need"; processed food for mass marketing; living on quick reading of the Word as opposed to a richer study that takes more time; something convenient but unhealthy for the long run.

FASTING: Abstinence from pleasure or food to set yourself apart for God.

FENCE: Protection; boundaries; "fenced in"; feeling trapped; offenses and other things hard to get over. See Deut 3:5.

FILES: Memory; proof; evidence; keeping records of wrongs. See 1 Cor 13:5.

FIRE: Passion for something; anointing; ministers; consumes the works of the flesh; baptism of fire; hell's fire judgment; anger (fiery temper, temper flare-ups); means for refining; Upper Room tongues of fire. See Matt 3:11, Heb 12:29, Ps 104:4, Acts 2:3.

FISHING: Evangelism ("fishers of men"); teaching in the world; put your line out (outreach); fishing for evidence; being lured or hooked. See Matt 4:19.

FLOATING UP: Getting a raise or promotion (spiritual or literal); giving up on a situation; becoming ungrounded.

FLOOR: Position of job or ministry; foundational structure; walking in secure or shaky situations (financial, governmental, national, home). See Matt 7:24.

FLOWERS: Beautiful; fragrant; lift you up; fragrance of the Lord; generational blessings (carry seeds); fading glory of man; express emotions (love, sympathy, concern). See Is 27:6,28:1.

FOOD: Spiritual nourishment; provision; fellowship; survival.

FOOTBALL: Your approach to an issue/situation (i.e., tackle it; punt decision); finding strategies to win souls; coach could be the Lord showing you the plays; teamwork is important; you will be tackled and pushed; could indicate a job, a court case, school, etc.

FREEZER: Storing spiritual food/teaching for a later time; emotionally frigid; frozen with fear of moving forward; deep

Page | 203

freeze (like a coma); extended time or extreme cold damages. See also *Refrigerator*.

FRONT: Future.

FURNACE: Bondage (i.e., iron furnace of Egypt); punishment; heat; source of warmth that may burn if touched. See Deut 4:20.

GATE: Access point; access needing permission or credentials. See Ps 100.

GIFT: Spiritual gifts; talents; anointing; something hidden to be unwrapped or revealed; generational gift or treasure; natural gifts you are born with; blessing. See Matt 25:14-30.

GRADUATION: Accomplishment; new beginning; end of an old season of testing and learning; time to go to work in the field

GRASS: Flesh; life; frailty; seasonal; maintenance. See Is 40:6.

GUN: Words with far-reaching impact; "shooting off your mouth"; authority (positive or negative); no bullets, then authority without power as a threat or bluff; protection; spiritual warfare; "stick to your guns" or don't back down; can kill destiny; deadline or "under the gun"; water gun–childish fighting; cap gun–cheap threat with no power.

HAMMER: Word of God; trying to "hammer things out"; weapon for bludgeoning. See Jer 23:29.

HONEY: Anointing; goodness; blessing; provision; sweet words; the Word of God to be desired more than honey. See Pro 24:13, Song of Sol 4:11, Ps 19:7-11.

HUNGER: Deprived of spiritual food and teaching; hunger and thirst after righteousness; a craving for something missing in life (good or bad).

ICE CREAM: Special treat; reward yourself; fun time; temporary pleasure (melts quickly); if consumed too quickly causes headaches; "I scream" (for something needed).

ICE WATER: Blessing; refreshing. See Pro 25:25.

IDOL: Strong delusion; something taking the place of God.

IMMOBILE: Fixed and firmly established; stillness (to know God); spiritual enemy is coming against you to hold you back or stop you. See 1 Chr 16:30, Ps 46:10.

IMMUNIZE: Redemption; blood of Jesus; create a resistance to temptation or sin; become unaffected by attacks; exempt. See Heb 9:11-12.

IMPLANT: Something planted; not original.

INCENSE: Prayers; worship and adoration at the altar; warning against burning incense to idols or other gods. See Jer 1:16, 44:3, Ez 8:11, 16:18, Ps 141:2.

INCEST: Spirit of perversion from you, the other person, or family.

INK: Scribe; writer; "mark" my words; tattoos. See Jer 36:2, 2 Cor 3:3, Lev 19:28.

INSECTS: Plague; small things that bug you; unclean; biting causes irritation. See Ex 8:24, 1 King 8:37, Is 7:18.

IRONING: Seared conscience; ironing problems out; correction; working out the wrinkles. See 1 Tim 4:2.

JEWELS: God's people; gifts of God; generational inheritance and prosperity; fake jewels–imitating the gifts of the Spirit, causes disappointment, has the sparkle, but no value or power.

JOG: Run the race set before you; "jog your memory". See Heb 12:1.

KARATE: Skilled protector; warrior; concentration; discipline; roots in Eastern mysticism. See 2 Cor 10:4.

KEYS: Spiritual authority; access; favor; answers. See Is 22:22, Matt 16:19.

KISS: Agreement; greeting; intimacy; deception/betrayal (Judas); seduction. See Luke 22:48.

KNIFE: Sharp, cutting words; division; self-defense; rightly divide the truth; surgical precision; betrayal (i.e., "knife in the back"); utility.

KNIT: Unity; joined together; new life knit in the womb. See Acts 10:11, Jud 20:11, Col 1:17.

LAMP: Light of God in us; God's Word; not to be hidden; insight. See Ps 119:105.

LATE: Timing issue; a warning that you could miss an appointed time God has for you.

LAUNDRY: Repentance; dealing with sin and issues; need for cleansing; clean up your act; "airing your dirty laundry" is displaying your mess in public.

LAVA: Destruction; eruption boiling over; judgment; creates path of destruction.

LAW: God's commandments; legalistic; Old Testament; man-made laws to create order and protection. See Josh 1:8.

LEAF: Healing; life or death cycle; seasons; people under leadership. See Ez 47:12, Rev 22:2.

LEAVEN: Doctrine of man kneaded into God's truth; corruption; flattery. See 1 Cor 5:6, Gal 5:9.

LEMON: Something went sour; bitter deal; can be a need for vitamin C; "make lemonade from lemons".

LILIES: Christ (Lily of the Valley); created beauty; white; fragrant; Easter lily–resurrection; Christians. See Song of Sol 2:1–2, Matt 6:28.

LOCK: Don't have access at this time; no access; blocked blessing; sealed and secure; protection; safety. See Song of Sol 4:12.

LOCKER: Store your identity/personal items.

LONG LINE: Patience; encourage you to wait; your time will come; leaving the line is giving up too soon; returning later to the end of the line is starting all over.

LOST: There is something important that you need to find; follow your path with the Lord's leading to your destination; misplaced.

LUGGAGE: Travel; if heavy, then lighten up; issues can be excess baggage; burdens.

MAIL: Nonverbal communication; incoming or outgoing message; junk mail–need to get rid of negative communication.

MAP: Direction; "mapping things out"; navigating the way; a plan; direction for life journey. See Jn 14:6.

MARBLE: Elegant but hard and cold (person or place).

MARBLES: Playing childish games; making an irrational decision (i.e., "have you lost your marbles?"); thoughts.

MARRIAGE: Covenant; vow; two becoming as one. See Heb 13:4, 1 Cor 7:2, Hos 2:19.

MEAT: Mature word and teaching. See Heb 5:14, 1 Cor 2:10.

MEDICINE: Need for healing; man's remedies verses God's; laughter is medicine for the soul.

MICROPHONE: Time to be heard; a larger audience; speak up.

MICROSCOPE: Magnified vision; seeing beyond the natural; vision for what is hidden; scrutinizes details under extreme magnification; spiritual sight to see what the natural eyes cannot.

MICROWAVE: Wanting things fast even if it's not the best.

MILK: Basics of the Word; lighter teaching (as opposed to the meat of the word); provision; food/teaching for infants or beginners. See 1 Pet 2:2, Heb 5:13.

MIRROR: Self-image; memory; reflect upon yourself/seeing what you were unaware of; vanity; another side of an issue looking back at you. See Jam 1:23.

MISCARRIAGE: Loss of something precious you have been anticipating; resolving pain from a past miscarriage; fear of miscarriage (does not usually mean literal miscarriage); aborting a plan or project that will not develop; something you are working on in an infant stage of development that fails to thrive.

MOLD: Storing up earthly treasures that will perish; something neglected too long; spiritual food not being used. See Matt 6:19.

MONEY: Favor of God; power; influence; authority; love of it is root of evil; the earth's currency to buy or sell; finding money–blessings will come unexpectedly. See also *Coins.*

MOVIE: Vision; seeing the big picture; spectator (rather than a participant in life); what you are watching.

MOVING: Literal moving; making a change from an old lifestyle; moving on to something new; salvation.

NAIL: Putting things together; piercing Jesus on the cross; "you nailed it". See Jn 19:16.

NAKED: Vulnerable; transparent; shame; seduction.

NEEDLE: A wordplay for "sowing" in the Spirit; mending others; creative work; stick you; "finding a needle in a haystack".

NEST: Family; empty nest–children moving out; investments.

NET: Evangelistic ministry (fishers of men); safety net to catch a fall from high places (i.e., prayer partner); financial net as a backup plan (i.e., insurance); trap; Internet. See Luke 5:4.

NEWS: Something you need to tune in to; information on past, current, or upcoming events; something new; the gospel is the Good News.

NEWSPAPER: Heralds information; worldly cares; headlines; promoting and advertising; local or international concerns.

OIL: Anointing; Holy Spirit; healing; blessing; slippery issues; reduces friction; helps things to work together smoothly.

OLD: Wisdom; antiques; a different time period; increased value; something getting old to you; outdated.

ORANGE (the fruit): A wordplay for "Son"-kissed; love of Jesus.

OVEN: Preparation; testing; judgment; refine (as gold).

PET: Something you have responsibility for; something precious to you; a pet issue.

PHOTOGRAPHS: Capture moments in time; visions; memories.

PILLOW: Rest; comfort; ease your mind/thoughts; what your thoughts keep resting on.

PLOW: Breaking new ground; pioneering the way; preparing to sow seed/the Word; groundbreaking.

PLUG (OUTLET): Power source; a place where you are "plugged in" or connected; resources.

POND: Community influence; "big fish in a small pond"; non-flowing.

PORK: Unclean; unsanctified meat; "pork belly" projects waste government tax money.

POTATOES: Staple/basic foundational teaching of the Word ("meat and potatoes"); growing hidden (in the ground); open your "eyes"; potato seed is called "true seed"; multiplies.

PREGNANT: New ministry, job, project developing; carrying a gift of God; something in the making that is about to come forth; expectations.

PUZZLE: Piecing things together (giving it a lot of thought); trying to see the bigger picture; problems; working out an issue (putting the pieces back together); hidden message.

QUILT: Comfort and security; different pieces or people coming together; generational blessing passed on.

RACE: Running the race set before you; competitive; life; "rat race"; hurriedness or urgency. See 1 Cor 9:24, Heb 12:1.

RAPE: Forced violation of your principles; defilement of boundaries and morals; forcefully asserting will upon others; controlling; to profane holy things; someone who cares only for themselves; abuse; forced reproduction. See Deut 22:25–28.

REFRIGERATOR: Preserving and storing spiritual nourishment (fulfilled or unfulfilled); keeping teaching fresh. See also *Freezer*.

REVERSE: Going backward; backing out of something; difficulty seeing your direction.

RHINESTONES: Counterfeit; cheap imitation of God's blessings; accepting less than God's best for you; showy costume jewelry; fake.

ROOF: Covering; protection; leader.

ROSE: Christ (Rose of Sharon); expression of love; fragrant and beautiful; sweet, refreshing to the spiritual senses; literally highly valued throughout the world. See Song of Sol 2:1.

SAND: Innumerable; humanity; descendants of Abraham; God's thoughts toward us; poor foundation; time; boundary; relaxing on the beach. See Gen 22:17, Job 29:18, Ps 139:17–18, Jer 5:22, Heb 11:11–12.

SAND CASTLES: Temporary; foolish (the foolish man built a house in the sand); foundation of man rather than Christ; washes away. See Matt 7:26.

SEED: Word of God; provision from; promise; faith; tithe. See Gen 1:29, Lev 27:30, 2 Chr 31:5, 1 Pet 1:23, Matt 12:31–32.

SHOWERING/BATHING: Cleansing outer toxins accumulated from day to day (i.e., words spoken, work issues); soaking in spiritual things.

SLOW MOTION: Things the enemy puts in your way to slow you down or stop you from moving into your calling; a time to slow down.

SMOKE: Glory (smoke filled the temple); offense ("smoke in your eyes"); sign of fire (spiritual or literal); method for concealment ("smoke screen"). See Is 6:4, Rev 15:8.

STOVE: A place for cooking up something; heart; preparation of spiritual food; a situation/issue that could be heating up; testing; trials; purification.

SWORD: The Bible; Word of God; armor of God. See Eph 6:17.

TABLE: Community; place of fellowship or agreement; gathering in a unit (i.e., family, church); "table the issue".

TAMBOURINE: Celebration; praise. See Ex 15:20, Ps 150:4, 2 Sam 6:5.

TELEPHONE: Communication; prophetic; hearing from someone or the Lord.

TELEVISION: Wordplay for "tell a vision"; prophetic vision; worldly communication; access into homes (good or bad).

TENNIS: Skill to serve; passing ideas back and forth; relationships (i.e., courting, score in love); involved in a racket or something dishonest.

TIRES: What your life or ministry rides on; carries you somewhere; Holy Spirit; bald tires–lack traction, are worn, and cause slipping; flat tire–not getting anywhere or in need of refreshment or refill. See Jn 3:8.

TOILET: Inner cleansing and healing; flushing things out of your life (i.e., toxic words or thoughts).

TOOLBOX: Carrying tools to fix problems; repertoire of abilities (i.e., résumé).

TOOTHBRUSH: Cleaning up your speech; "brushing up" on something. See Pro 16:24.

TOPLESS: Ability to nurture; freedom from restraint; vulnerable; getting something "off your chest."

TOWEL: Humility and servanthood (as in washing feet).

TRASH: Cleaning up some things in life; getting rid of things in your mind and heart.

TREASURE: Heart (where your treasure is, your heart is also) riches; Kingdom of Heaven; favor; wisdom and knowledge. See Matt 6:20–21, 13:44, Col 2:3.

TREES: Leaders; people; branching out; family tree– generational issues (positive or negative); olive tree–anointing; fruit tree bearing ripe fruit–successful leadership that reproduces itself; leaves for the healing of the nations; oaks of righteousness; tree cut down–a fallen leader; stump–hope for restoration in time (i.e., Nebuchadnezzar). See Is 61:3, Ps 1:3, Dan 4:23, Zech 4:12.

TRUMPET: Herald the return of Christ; Feast of Trumpets; victory; warning ("sound the alarm"); impending judgment; resurrection of the dead; last call; Jericho fell; angels gather

His elect. See Ez 33:1–6, Num 10:1-10, Lev 23:24, Jos 6:20, Joel 2:15, Matt 24:31, 1 Cor 15:52, 1 Thes 4:16.

UMBRELLA: Protective spiritual or natural covering; oversized can cover a large group; could be blocking teaching and refreshing.

URINATE OPENLY: Relieving a situation publicly; ridding of toxins; inner cleansing; rebellion; defilement; offensive actions; disrespectful.

VACUUM: Remove accumulated sin (i.e., bad attitude, sins, unforgiveness); deliverance; repentance; maintenance of cleaning in your life and heart; isolation; void of air/spirit.

VINE: Jesus, the Vine; jobs and opportunities; heard through the grapevine/rumors; Israel. See Jn 15:5.

VINEGAR: Reproach; bitterness; acidic; fermented; sour; preserves things; cleaner; aids digestion; pickling. See Ruth 2:14, Luke 23:36.

VIOLIN: Praise; joy; peace; "fiddling around"; soothing; serenade of love; melodious. See Ps 150:4, Is 38:20.

VOLLEYBALL: Passing ideas back and forth.

VOMIT: Purging something from your life; physically or spiritually infected by negative influences; repeating the behavior after forgiveness has been obtained is like a dog returning to his own vomit. See Pro 26:11.

WALLET: Carries your identity; money; authority for card use and access to places (i.e., gym, library); stolen–enemy has unauthorized access to your information and finances; lost–you lose sight of your identity and purpose.

WALLS: Boundaries; divisions; can have watchman who provides warnings; to "hit a wall" is to be at a standstill; "walled in" is confined; "walled off" is restricted access; "off the wall" is something unusual and non-traditional; "wall of protection."

WATER: Spiritual condition; doctrines; size of the body of water related to size of influence (e.g., a huge lake could indicate a megachurch and a pond could indicate a small church); flooding is being overwhelmed (in a good or negative way); "trying to keep your head above water"; cold or hot spiritually; ice water–cool conditions, refreshing; boiling–something reaching the boiling point in your life, anger. See Is 11:9, Mark 9:41, Jn 1:31.

WEAPON: Warfare; protection; ready to fight; take a stand; prepare with the Word of God (sword). See Gen 49:5, Neh 4:16–18, 2 Cor 10:4.

WINDOW: Vision to see; revelation; open window of blessing; partial vision (see through a glass darkly). See Mal 3:10, 1 Cor 13:12.

WINE: Holy Communion; teaching; Holy Spirit is the new wine; drunkard is unwise; be sober; wineskins/flesh (old or new). See Is 5:22, Pro 20:1, 21:17, Mark 2:22, 14:23, Acts 2:4, 1 Pet 5:8, Eph 5:18.

WOOD: Flesh; humanity; compassion; building from earthly or natural materials.

WORK OUT: Resolve issues; discipline; build strength.

X-RAY: Discernment; reveals what is hidden; get an inside look to detect the presence of defects; vision that sees through the flesh.

YEARBOOK: Reviewing the past; personal history.

YEAST: Sin; hypocrisy; fluffed up; flattery; pride; Christianity fermented with modern teachings. See Matt 16:6.

YELLING: Something you need to hear; trying to get your attention; issuing a warning.

YO-YO: Emotional ups and downs; busy but getting nowhere.

ZIPPER: Uniting; bringing together; "zip it up" or "zip your lip."

ABOUT THE AUTHOR

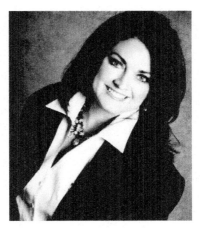

Terri Meredith has served in various levels of ministry spanning over thirty years. She is a conference speaker, Bible teacher, mentor, and has appeared on television and radio. She currently serves in ministries including altar care, dream interpretation, and women's street ministry. She also has a BS degree in Education. She is a wife, mother, and proud grandmother.

AUTHOR'S ACKNOWLEDGMENTS

My deepest appreciation and heartfelt thanks goes out to my dear friend Dr. Jennifer Minigh, owner of ShadeTree Publishing. Without her help, this book would not have been written. She offered her support, time, and tremendous insight into scripture, writing, and dreams. She has such a beautiful gift and heart. Truly, thank you.

I would also like to thank the following people, because without their help, this book would still be a dream:

A special thanks to my daughter Heather May, of Heather May Photography, for designing the front and back book cover art. Your work is greatly appreciated.

I would also like to thank Beth Stewart of Beth Stewart Ministries for being a constant source of encouragement. Also to my husband and son, for their love and support through the writing process.

Thanks to Apostle Jane Hamon for reviewing the manuscript and sharing some of her dream stories and advice.

I respectfully acknowledge the work of the late John Paul Jackson for his pioneering efforts in Christian dream interpretation, forging through the complexities of dreaming and always teaching with humility and integrity. My condolences to his family.

Finally, thank you to all those who have taught, researched, and shared their information on dreams. To name a few: Michael French, Ira Milligan, Jane Hamon, Barbie Breathitt, James Goll, and Jim Driscoll.

REVIEW REQUEST

I hope you have gained some helpful knowledge from *Dreams Revealed* about dream interpretation.

Now that you've read this book, if you enjoyed it, then please let other readers know. Let's share the knowledge and help people.

SCRIPTURES AND REFERENCES

[1] Jackson, John Paul. "The Mystery of Dreams." Dreams and Mysteries. Daystar. 17 Oct. 2014. Television.

[2] "Brain Basics: Understanding Sleep." National Institute of Neurological Disorders and Stroke (NINDS). 2007. Accessed May 7, 2015. http://www.ninds.nih.gov/disorders/brain_basics/understanding_sleep.htm#dreaming.

[3] "REM Sleep." REM Sleep. Accessed May 7, 2015. http://www.bettersleep.org/better-sleep/stages-of-sleep/rem-sleep/#sthash.nBAnS0CQ.dpuf.

[4] Jacob Empson and Michael B. Wang. Sleep and Dreaming. 3rd ed. Houndmills, Basingstoke, Hampshire: Palgrave, 2002.

[5] Wilse Webb. "Physiological Dream Research." Britannica.com. Accessed May 7, 2015. http://britannica.com/EB checked/topic/171188/dream/38755/physiological-dream-research.

[6] "REM Sleep." REM Sleep. Accessed May 7, 2015. http://www.bettersleep.org/better-sleep/stages-of-sleep/rem-sleep/#sthash.nBAnS0CQ.dpuf.

[7] M.R. Trimble, "What Happens When We Sleep?—HowStuffWorks." HowStuffWorks. 198. Accessed May 7, 2015. http://health.howstuffworks.com/mental-health/sleep/basics/what-happens-when-we-sleep.htm.

[8] U. Voss, R. Holzmann, I. Tuin, J.A. Hobson., Lucid dreaming: a state of consciousness with features of both waking and non-lucid dreaming. Sleep. 2009 Sep;32(9):1191–200.

[9] "How Much Sleep Do We Really Need?" National Sleep Foundation. 2015. Accessed May 7, 2015. http://sleepfoundation.org/how-sleep-works/how-much-sleep-do-we-really-need.

[10] "Lack of Sleep Is Affecting Americans, Finds the National Sleep Foundation." National Sleep Foundation. Accessed May 7, 2015. http://sleepfoundation.org/media-center/press-release/lack-sleep-affecting-americans-finds-the-national-sleep-foundation.

[11] D.F. Kripke, L. Garfinkel, D.L. Wingard, M.R. Klauber, M.R. Marler. Mortality associated with sleep duration and insomnia. Arch Gen Psychiatry. 2002;59:131-6.

[12] "Sleep Disorder Statistics." Accessed May 7, 2015. http://www.stasticbrain.com. http://www.statisticbrain.com/sleeping-disorder-statistics/.

[13] Maureen Mackey, "Sleepless in America: A $32.4 Billion Business." *The Fiscal Times*. 2012. Accessed May 7, 2015. http://www.thefiscaltimes.com/Articles/2012/07/23/Sleepless-in-America-A-32-4-Billion-Business.

[14] "Lack of Sleep Is Affecting Americans, Finds the National Sleep Foundation." - National Sleep Foundation. Accessed May 7, 2015. http://sleepfoundation.org/media-center/press-release/lack-sleep-affecting-americans-finds-the-national-sleep-foundation.

[15] "Best Time of Day to Do Anything." Best Time of Day to Do Anything. Accessed May 7, 2015. http://www.totalhealthnutritioncenter.com/pages/Best-Time-of-Day-to-do-Anything.html.

[16] C.G. Jung, and R. F. C. Hull. "Psychology and Religion: West and East." In *The Collected Works of C.G. Jung*. New ed. Vol. 11. London: Routledge & Kegan Paul, 1971.

[17] C.G. Jung, and R. F. C. Hull. "Psychology and Religion: West and East." In *The Collected Works of C.G. Jung*. New ed. Vol. 11. London: Routledge & Kegan Paul, 1971.

[18] Jeremiah 29:8–9

[19] Ecclesiastes 5:3 KJV

[20] Matthew 6:21

[21] 1 Peter 5:8

[22] Matthew 13:25

[23] James 4:8

[24] "Twelve Famous Dreams: Creativity and Famous Discoveries from Dreams." Brilliant Dreams. Accessed May 7, 2015. http://brilliantdreams.com/product/famous-dreams.htm.

[25] 1 Corinthians 2:14 NIV

[26] Joel 2:28

[27] Luke 12:48

[28] Joel 2:28

[29] Ephesians 5:20

[30] Revelation 12:10

[31] Jeremiah 29:11

[32] Job 32:8, 33:4

[33] John 7:38–39

[34] John 3:8

[35] Isaiah 28:16; 1 Peter 2:6

[36] John 6:35

[37] Matthew 25:1–10; Mark 2:19–20; John 3:29

[38] Zechariah 13:1
[39] Hebrews 6:20
[40] 1 Corinthians 3:11; Isaiah 28:16
[41] 1 Corinthians 10:4
[42] John 10:7–9
[43] John 4:10
[44] Colossians 1:18
[45] Revelation 5:6; John 1:36
[46] John 1:14; Revelation 19:13
[47] John 11:25, 14:6
[48] Revelation 5:5
[49] Luke 1:70
[50] John 14:6
[51] Matthew 21:42; 1 Peter 2:4
[52] Revelation 3:14
[53] 2 Peter 1:9; Revelation 22:16
[54] John 15:1
[55] John 10:7-9
[56] John 14:6
[57] John 11:25
[58] Revelation 1:8, 22:13
[59] Song of Solomon 2:1
[60] Song of Solomon 2:1
[61] Luke 1:69
[62] Isaiah 4:2
[63] John 8:12, 9:5
[64] Matthew 13:45
[65] Matthew 13:24
[66] Matthew 13:31
[67] Matthew 13:44
[68] Matthew 13:47
[69] Jeremiah 4:7
[70] Psalm 10:9
[71] "Parable". 2015. In Merriam-Webster.com. Retrieved April 28, 2015, from http://www.merriam-webster.com/dictionary/parable.
[72] Proverbs 25:2
[73] Esther 1:6, 8:15; Exodus 25; Numbers 4:6, 15:38; Jeremiah 10:9; Ezekiel 23:6, 27:7, 24
[74] Exodus 25–28, 35-36, 38–39; Numbers 4:13; 2 Chronicles 2:7,14, 3:14; Judges 8:26; Esther 1:6, 8:15; Song of Solomon 3:10; Mark 15:17,20; John 19:2, 5; Proverbs 31:22; Jeremiah 10:9; Song of Solomon 7:5; Ezekiel 27:7, 16; Luke 16:19; Acts 16:14; Revelation 17:4, 18:12, 16

[75] 1 John 1:5–7
[76] Matthew 10:30
[77] Psalm 147:4
[78] Proverbs 27:17

NOTES